JET Library

Joint Education & Training Library

Occupational Voice Loss

Occupational Voice Loss

Nerys Williams
University of Birmingham
Birmingham, United Kingdom

Paul Carding
Freeman Hospital
Newcastle-upon-Tyne, United Kingdom

With contributions by
Erkki Vilkman and Jeremy Freedman

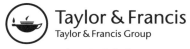

Taylor & Francis
Taylor & Francis Group

Boca Raton   London   New York   Singapore

Published in 2005 by
Taylor & Francis Group
6000 Broken Sound Parkway NW, Suite 300
Boca Raton, FL 33487-2742

International Standard Book Number-10: 0-8247-2877-7 (Hardcover)
International Standard Book Number-13: 978-0-8247-2877-9 (Hardcover)

Library of Congress Cataloging-in-Publication Data

Catalog record is available from the Library of Congress

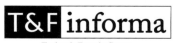

Taylor & Francis Group
is the Academic Division of T&F Informa plc.

**Visit the Taylor & Francis Web site at
http://www.taylorandfrancis.com**

Foreword

This book presents a cohesive compilation of current information about the causes, impact, prevention, legal standing, diagnosis, and treatment of occupation-related voice disorders. Even though voice clinicians have long noticed that certain professions appear to have a higher incidence of voice problems, it is only somewhat recently that actual data has been available to show that occupation can be a significant risk factor for voice disorders. Such formal recognition has been coupled with a growing international interest in developing occupational health standards for voice use, similar to other standards that have already been developed in various countries for workplace-related factors such as noise exposure, air quality, etc. Thus, the publication of this book is quite timely and should have a positive impact on efforts to improve vocal health.

The production of voice is a truly remarkable phenomenon. When one hears the voice of a professional singer or accomplished public speaker, it is hard to imagine that the full rich sound originates as the vibration of laryngeal (vocal folds) tissue that is no more than a few millimeters thick. Yet even though vocal fold tissue appears thin and delicate, it is unique in the human body for its requirement to withstand the cyclic generation of collision and shearing forces at high repetition rates (generally in the range of 100 to 300 times per second for normal speaking) during its normal function to produce voice. Added to the mechanical demands on vocal fold tissue is the fact that the larynx also sits at the junction of the pulmonary and digestive systems, serving as the main "sentry" to protect the lower airways and lungs from foreign bodies. In this location, the delicate tissues of the vocal folds are quite susceptible to both the refluxing of (digestion-related) acidic materials from the esophagus, and to any airborne irritants (unhumidified air, pollutants, etc.) that are inspired by the lungs. Damage to vocal fold tissue results when an individual's tolerances for mechanical trauma and/or environmental irritation are exceeded, perhaps related to occupational demands. Normal laryngeal voice production can also be heavily challenged by psychological state (e.g., work-related emotional stress), both directly in terms of increasing laryngeal muscle tension and mechanical trauma of vocal fold tissues, and indirectly by leading to detrimental increases in environmental irritants.

The laryngeal production of voice is but one important component of the human speech production apparatus, which also includes the articulatory structures (tongue, jaw, soft palate, lips) and pulmonary system. A disruption in the function of any of these structures can cause a speech communication disorder. However, given the high mechanical demands and environmental challenges consistently placed on the larynx during normal speech production, it is perhaps not surprising that the larynx is the component in the speech production system that is by far the most susceptible to use-related "break down." It is becoming increasingly clear that occupation can be a major determinant of how an individual uses his/her voice on a daily basis. Thus, this book's major focus on the role of occupation in voice disorders is appropriate and well placed.

The variety of specialties represented by the authors of this book is an accurate reflection of the need for occupational voice disorders to be managed by an interdisciplinary team. Such interdisciplinary involvement is equally critical to the design of future research efforts aimed at gaining a more complete understanding of the complex interrelationships between occupation, voice use and voice disorders. This book should not only serve as a valuable clinical resource, but its organization should also help structure and direct new investigations into the role of occupation in voice problems.

Robert E. Hillman, Ph.D., CCC-SLP
Co-Director and Research Director
Center for Laryngeal Surgery and
Voice Rehabilitation,
Massachusetts General Hospital,
and Associate Professor in Surgery
and Health Sciences and Technology,
Harvard Medical School, Boston,
Massachusetts, U.S.A.

Preface

The human voice is a complex structure without which most of us would struggle daily. Yet we spend little time or effort in ensuring it works to maximum efficiency and barely notice our voices unless we get a cold. Then we know how unpleasant it is to be hoarse and to find speech painful and how difficult it can be to communicate. The importance of avoiding voice problems cannot be overemphasized, yet many jobs and occupations carry the potential for causing voice problems due to design or working conditions.

Relatively little has been written about the relationship between work and voice health so we hope that this book will stimulate further research to fill the gaps in our knowledge. We also hope we will provide those with an interest in the occupational aspects of voice use with information, tools and suggested approaches to identifying hazards to vocal health, controlling risks from the work environment and educating workers about how they can contribute to ensuring that one of their best assets remains healthy.

Nerys Williams
Paul Carding

Acknowledgments

I would like to thank my parents, Dilys and Glyn, and my brother David for nothing in particular and everything in general. To Neil for putting up with my working whilst on holiday and to those "models" who helped with the photographs; Steve, Jenny, Ching, Paul, Lorraine, Ali and Lorraine again.

Nerys Williams

I would like to thank Kate, my wife, for all of her support and understanding. The book is dedicated to my children, James and Jenny; they may read it and understand it one day! Finally, I would like to thank my patients who continue to report individual insights and dilemmas which continually challenge my thoughts and opinions.

Paul Carding

Contents

1

How the Human Voice Is Produced

VOICE AND SPEECH

When a human being speaks, the listener hears the product of both the voice and the speech articulators. *Voice* is made essentially by the vibration of the vocal folds (this is called "phonation"). However, as we shall see, the sound that radiates out of the mouth is far more complex than this vibration because it is modified and resonated by the rest of the vocal tract to produce a recognizable voice quality. Furthermore, the articulatory structures of the vocal tract (including the lips, tongue, and soft palate) shape the sound source in an infinite number of combinations to make *speech*. This coordination of phonatory and articulatory behaviors represents arguably the most advanced sensori-motor system to be found in the human body (1).

Speech and voice require precise coordination of intricate muscle movements executed with accuracy and speed. The physiological flexibility of the vocal tract and the anatomical variations among different people allow for an enormous range of normal voice and speech qualities. This means that individual speakers may alter their own laryngeal and oropharyngeal structures to change their own voice quality. This could be a conscious act (for example, in the case of an actor or impersonator) or an unconscious change (for example, as a result of vocal fatigue or postural tension). This fact has implications for how we assess and measure components of speech and voice for diagnostic purposes (2). (These issues will be discussed in a later chapter). This chapter focuses on the main features of human voice and how it is made.

HOW VOICE IS MADE

All physical sounds are made by a force of energy that "excites" a source of vibration. This vibration results in the generation of a sound waveform that, in turn, is resonated in the connecting "resonator" structures. In the case of human voice, the vocal folds, working together, constitute a vibrator that is activated by the excitor—the exhaled air. The pharyngeal, naso-pharyngeal, and oral spaces (the "supra-glottic vocal tract") resonate the sound as it passes through on its way out of the mouth.

Figure 1 consists of two line drawings of an endoscopic view of the vocal folds—one in adducted and one in abducted position. The illustration is carefully labeled to denote the vocal folds, arytenoid cartilages, ary-epiglottic folds, "false vocal folds," and glottic space.

The Vocal Structures "at Rest"

When the larynx is at rest and respiration is quiet, the vocal folds remain essentially open to facilitate unimpeded airflow in and out of the lungs. Detailed observation does detect minor vocal fold opening ("abduction") on quiet inspiration and slight closing ("adduction") on quiet expiration. Similarly,

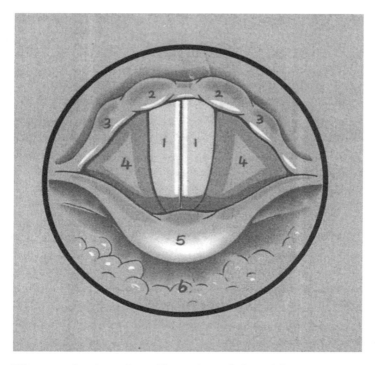

Figure 1 Anterior. Posterior, left, right orientation. (From Berkovitz and Moxham, A Textbook of Head and Neck Anatomy, 1988, Figs. 133 and 134.)

the whole larynx moves slightly up and down in sympathy with the outflow and inflow of respiratory air (3). In forceful inspiration (i.e., when taking a "big breath in"), the folds are drawn wide apart to a position of full abduction to allow maximum air input.

How the Voice Starts

Immediately prior to phonation, the vocal folds open rapidly to allow an intake of air (4). Then, as the airflow begins to expire, the lateral crico-arytenoid muscles contract to bring the vocal folds together in the midline. As the pulmonic air (air from the lungs) is exhaled, it meets resistance at the level below the "closed" vocal folds. This "subglottic air pressure" increases until it reaches a level which overcomes the vocal fold resistance and they peel apart from their inferior border. When the vocal folds finally separate at their superior margin, a puff of air is released. The resulting negative pressure results in the vocal folds closing rapidly again as they are sucked back together. The cycle then repeats. Contact between the vocal folds increases until the subglottic air pressure is high enough to blow the vocal folds apart again. Rapid repetition of this cycle produces the vibration that we hear as the "vocal sound."

The Normal Vibratory Cycle

For voice to be produced, the vocal folds need to repeatedly vibrate in a cycle of closing and opening phases (5). Depending on the frequency ("pitch") of the voice, this will usually be happening hundreds of times per second. In normal voice, the closing phase of the vocal folds is more rapid than the opening phase.

The two vocal folds have to be structurally and functionally symmetrical in order to vibrate symmetrically. Similarly the vocal folds need to be at the same anatomical level to each other ("on plane"), and must have sufficient elasticity to close rapidly in order to produce an efficient and effective vibrating system. When all of these conditions are met (i.e., in the normal healthy larynx), then a clear voice can be initiated and maintained (6). In general, the inter-arytenoid muscles adduct the cartilaginous portion of both vocal folds and hold them together while the anterior portion of each fold is gently adducted but free to vibrate in the expiratory airflow. Full vocal fold adduction during phonation has traditionally been regarded as the norm. However, various studies suggest that there are wide variations of "normal" glottal configurations (7,8), as well as common differences between sexes and age groups (9,10).

INDIVIDUAL DIFFERENCES IN VOICE QUALITY

The individuality of a person's speech and voice are the product of the organic and phonetic features of the speaker (11). Organic factors are derived from the nature of the speaker's individual anatomical apparatus and their relationship with each other. This includes the dimensions and geometry of the nasal, oral, pharyngeal, and laryngeal structures, as well as function of the respiratory system. Phonetic features refer to the speaker's habitual use of the speaking and voicing apparatus. The specific combination of a person's anatomical configuration and his/her habitual physiology results in a voice that is unique to each individual. This explains why listening to voice and speech quality enables us to distinguish between one speaker and another.

The *frequency* of the glottal signal is a result of the number of vibratory cycles per second (measured in hertz). The rate of vibration of the vocal folds is a function of the vocal fold length, elasticity, tension, and mass, and their subsequent resistance to subglottal air pressure (12). The maintenance of a steady vocal frequency requires control of all of these interacting physiological features. Frequency increases with a lengthening of the vocal folds and the subsequent thinning and stiffening of the vocalis muscles (13). Considerable normative data of habitual speaking pitch or speaking fundamental frequency exists (12), although there is a huge range of what is considered "normal" depending on the age, sex, emotional state, communicative intent, mood, and personality of the speaker. Similarly there are data on vocal pitch range both in terms of maximum range and habitual speaking range (12).

Vocal loudness is the perceptual correlate of *amplitude*— the size of the oscillation of the vocal folds. The amplitude of these vibrations is largely determined by the force of the transglottal airflow. Increasing both the airflow through the larynx and the vocal fold resistance (and subsequent subglottal pressure) will result in an increase in vocal loudness. Like vocal frequency, there are data on normal vocal intensity (habitual and range) in a variety of settings (12).

Changes in the shape of the whole vocal tract (the oral, nasal, pharyngeal, and laryngeal cavities) and the dimensions of each cavity relative to one another can be achieved in numerous ways. For example, protruding the lips, retracting the tongue base, lowering the larynx, or lowering the soft palate will all dramatically alter the sound of the resultant voice. Furthermore, the supralaryngeal tract acts as a resonating chamber for the complex acoustic signal generated by the vibrating vocal folds. The specific geometry and dimensions of an individual speaker's vocal tract will determine the "timbre" or resonating properties of the voice. Skilled speakers and singers learn to manipulate these oral, nasal, and pharyngeal structures to maximize their resonant properties. This is not an easy thing to do because vocal resonance will, of course, continually change as we speak (i.e., change vocal pitch or intensity, articulate different sounds). *Oral resonance* is affected by the degree of jaw movement, mouth opening, tongue body raising, and pharyngeal constriction. *Nasal resonance* is affected by excessive or too limited action of the velopharyngeal sphincter during speech (or some degree of nasal obstruction). The final result is a sound with an appropriate oral/nasal balance. Appropriate oral/nasal resonance is not only necessary for normal sounding speech and voice, but is important to facilitate good voice projection and vocal efficiency.

OTHER FEATURES OF THE HUMAN VOICE

It is important to recognize that a voice is more than just a physiological act or just the result of a set of muscular movements. For example, the skilled listener can acquire considerable information about speakers from the way they use speech rhythm and vocal intonation. These "paralinguistic features" of voice (14) represent an immensely powerful means of conveying intent, mood, and personality. Our speech and voice may also provide (either intentionally or unintentionally) messages about our education, social status, emotional state, and personality. It is rare for speakers to use these features consciously unless they are vocal performers or have had extensive voice training. More common is the unconscious use of these features—and therefore they may be more revealing than the speaker intended. This is the basis for the phrase "it's not what you say, it's the way that you say it."

Speech rhythm can be specific to a language and even an accent. Speech rhythm (and stress) is one of the most difficult linguistic features for foreign speakers to master. Truly bi-lingual speakers who were exposed to several speech rhythm patterns from birth do not appear to have this problem. Loss of natural speech rhythms (for example, in some neurologically impaired speakers) can result in almost unintelligible speech. *Speech rate* is likely to reflect our state of arousal (excited, drowsy, stressed, etc.) and is clearly linked to other physiological systems such as pulse and respiratory rate (14). Our speech rate is often interpreted as an indicator of anxiety (if it is too fast) or low intellect (if it is too slow) (15). Vocal *intonation* refers to varying vocal pitch to indicate communicative intent (e.g., to ask a question or to indicate a statement) and to manipulate conversation (e.g., to encourage a response or to indicate that you have not finished speaking). *Pitch range* may reflect emotional status: a wide range may indicate excitability; a narrow ("flatter") range may be interpreted as sadness or impassiveness (16). Habitually high pitch may indicate anxiety and low pitch may suggest (or at least give the impression of) depression (17). A speaker's *vocal quality* may also reflect the emotional content of his/her verbal message (18). For example, a breathy vocal quality may indicate anxiety (19) or vulnerability (20). Conversely, a "creaky" low-pitched voice may indicate a relaxed state and even higher social status (21). Vocal *loudness* appears to be different between the sexes: men talk more loudly than women (21). Not surprisingly, we commonly associate vocal loudness with confidence and an extroverted personality (22). It could, of course, also indicate a lack of the speaker's awareness of the environment (i.e., in a library or church) or, commonly, could suggest hearing problems.

A comprehensive understanding of how the human voice is made provides a physiological explanation of these paralinguistic features of voice. It should, of course, be remembered that the interpretation of these features in a particular speaker is subjective and may vary from one listener to another. However, understanding these aspects of voice enables us to appreciate why a voice-disordered person may describe severe levels of personal disability and distress (23,24).

REFERENCES

1. Fawcus R. Chapter 1. In: Freeman M, Fawcus M, eds. Voice Disorders and Their Management. London: Whurr Publishers, 2000.

2. Carding PN. Measuring the Effectiveness of Voice Therapy. London: Whurr, 2000.

3. Tucker H. The Larynx. New York: Thième, 1993.

4. Wyke B. Recent advances in the neurology of phonation and reflex mechanisms in the larynx. Br J Disord Commun 1967; 2:2–14.

5. Hirano M, Bless DM. Videostroboscopic Examination of the Larynx. London: Whurr, 1993.

6. Woo P, Colton R, Casper J, Brewer D. Diagnostic value of stroboscopic examination in hoarse patients. J Voice 1991; 5:231–238.

7. Murry T, Xu JJ, Woodson GE. Glottal configuration associated with fundamental frequency and vocal register. J Voice 1998; 12:44–49.

8. Gelfer MP, Bultemeyer DK. Evaluation of vocal fold vibratory patterns in normal voices. J Voice 1990; 4:335–345.

9. Biever DM, Bless DM. Vibratory characteristics of the vocal folds in young adult and geriatric women. J Voice 1989; 3:120–131.

10. Sodersten M, Hertegard S, Hammarberg B. Glottal closure, transglottal airflow and voice quality in healthy middle-aged women. J Voice 1995; 9:182–197.

11. Laver J. The Phonetic Description of Voice Quality. Cambridge: Cambridge University Press, 1980.

12. Baken RJ, Orlikoff RE. Clinical Measurement of Speech and Voice. 2nd ed. San Diego: Singular, 2000.

13. Harris T, Harris S, et al. The Voice Clinic Handbook. London: Whurr, 2000.

14. Mathieson L. Greene and Mathieson's The Voice and Its Disorders. 6th ed. London: Whurr, 2001.

15. Ryan EB, Giles H, Sebastian RJ. An integrative perspective for the study of attitudes towards language variation. In: Ryan EB, Giles H, eds. The Social Psychology of Language. London: Edward Arnold, 1982.

16. Scherer K. Expression of emotion in voice and music. J Voice 1995; 9:235–248.

17. Moses PJ. The Voice of Neurosis. New York: Grune and Stratton, 1954.

18. White A, Deary IJ, Wilson JA. Psychiatric disturbance and personality traits in dysphonic patients. Eur J Disord Commun 1997; 32:307–314.

19. Gudykunst WB. Intergroup communication. In: Giles, ed. The Social Psychology of Language and Communication Studies. London: Edward Arnold, 1986.

20. Freeman M, Fawcus M. Voice Disorders and Their Management. London: Whurr, 2000.

21. Scherer K, Giles H. Social Markers in Speech. Cambridge: Cambridge University Press, 1979.

22. Street RL, Hopper R. A model of speech style evaluation. In: Ryan EB, Giles H, eds. The Social Psychology of Language. London: Edward Arnold, 1982.

23. Ramig LO, Verdolini K. Treatment efficacy: voice disorders. J Speech, Lang Hear Res 1998; 41:S101–S166.

24. Wilson JA, Deary IJ, Millar A, MacKenzie K. The quality of life impact of dysphonia. Clin Otolaryngol. In press.

2

Occupational Groups at Risk of Voice Disorders

It has been suggested that some groups of workers are more at risk of such disorders than others. This chapter reviews the published research on groups at risk.

BACKGROUND

Studies in the United States estimate that approximately 25% of the American working population considers its voice as critical to job performance (1). Therefore, for a large section of the working population, the prevention of occupational voice disorders is essential. Comparable figures have been reported in Finland (2), but data are not available for the United Kingdom or Europe as a whole; however, there is no reason to believe that a smaller proportion of the United Kingdom and European workers are not similarly dependent on adequate voice and speech.

PREVALENCE OF VOICE DISORDERS IN THE GENERAL AND WORKING POPULATIONS

Within the general population of the United States, various studies have reported that between 3% and 9% of people will report a voice abnormality at any one time (3). Other work on the background prevalence of voice disorder in the general population has suggested rates varying between 0.65% (4) and 15% (5). In 1952, Morely (4) reported a study based solely on a student population with the finding of a low prevalence rate; this could have been due to either the low frequency of the condition or the young age of the respondents. Similarly, Laguaite's (5) study included elderly subjects and so, again, is not directly comparable to studies based strictly on working populations. Laguaite looked at the frequency of diagnosis depending on whether it was the opinion of an expert (found in 7% of the cases) or a self-reported voice problem (15% of the cases). As a higher prevalence of voice problems has previously been reported in the elderly (6), the inclusion of elderly subjects in Laguaite's study may also have been a factor in finding higher rates of symptoms. We can, therefore, conclude from the published research that self-reported voice disorders are common in the general population and occur in both young and old people. Indeed, the work of Coyle et al. (7) found that retired persons and homemakers were two of the most common "occupations" presenting to voice clinics.

Occupational Groups at Risk

For some groups of workers, voice impairment can be employment threatening, as some jobs cannot be performed without adequate vocal capacity.

Certain groups such as teachers and singers have been studied extensively and have been reported to have higher frequencies of voice disorders than the general population (8).

There are two main studies that have looked at wider occupational groupings.

Both a Swedish (9) and an American (10) study attempted to establish the relative frequency of various occupations attending voice clinics and compare them to the general population. They made the presumption that a greater representation of a particular occupation in the clinical caseload meant a greater risk for the occupation to cause an occupational voice disorder.

In the Swedish study, Fritzell (9) examined 1,212 patients of working age, who were attending eight voice clinics across the country over a 6-month period between 1992 and 1993.

In the American study, Titze et al. (10) identified 174 adults attending two voice clinics between 1991 and 1993.

In both studies, the frequency of symptoms in a particular occupational group was determined and compared to the number of overall workers in the country reported to be working with that job title. The results are shown in Table 1.

When the results of the two studies were combined they suggested that the occupation "singer" was at greatest risk of voice disorder. Singers were followed by counselors/social workers, teachers, lawyers, clergy, salespersons, ticket reservation/travel agents, and, interestingly, health care workers. Of particular interest was the subgroup of "salespersons"—that of telesales or salespersons—as it is this group of people

Table 1 Pooled Results from United States and Swedish Studies on Occupations at Risk of Voice Disorders

	% in population	% of clinic attendees
Salespersons	13	10
Subgroup telesales	0.78	2.3
Factory workers	14.5	5.6
Clerical workers	10.6	8.6
Teachers	4.2	19.6
Counsellors	0.19	1.6
Singers	0.02	11.5

Source: From Ref. 8.

whose employment is most likely to contain the tasks performed in call center environments, a growing employer of workers across the world.

While a high frequency of voice disorders in singers is relevant, they represent only a small group of the working population. The most disturbing findings from the public health perspective are those occupations which employ large numbers of workers. "Teacher" was the most common "at risk" occupation attending the clinics and, across the two studies, was four times more commonly represented clinically than in the population at large.

Teachers

The reported prevalence of voice problems in teachers depends on whether the diagnosis is based on objectively diagnosed vocal cord pathology or on subjective symptoms. Studies have reported prevalence rates of 4.4% (11) and 90% (12).

Smith et al. (13) analyzed 242 responses from primary and secondary teachers in the United States and compared the frequency of voice problems with those of individuals in other occupations. They found that teachers were more likely to have a voice problem (15% vs. 6%) when asked about ten specific voice symptoms and five physical symptoms of discomfort. They found that:

- 47.5% of teachers complained of hoarseness compared to 21.3% of controls. Teachers averaged almost two symptoms compared to none in other occupations.
- 20% of teachers but 0% of nonteachers reported resultant time lost from work.
- 4.2% of teachers said that the voice problem was significant enough for them to consider a change of occupation.

Similar findings were found in a study by Russell et al. (14) in Australian teachers. Sapir et al. (15) confirmed the findings regarding work capability in a study that found that more than one-third of teachers with voice problems missed work as a result.

Different types of teaching places different demands on voice. An American study by Smith et al. (16) looked at 924 teachers and found that of the 554 teachers who replied to the survey, more than 38% reported that teaching had negatively affected their voice and 39% reported having difficulty with teaching lessons because of voice problems. Female teachers reported more frequently than male teachers (38% vs. 26% respectively, $p < 0.05$), both acute ($p < 0.05$) and chronic ($p < 0.05$) voice problems. There were no gender differences in the perception that a voice problem adversely affected their current or future teaching career. Females had a higher probability of reporting voice problems compared to men (odds ratio 1.7–2.1). Teaching physical education presented the highest risk of voice disorder, independent of gender, hours of teaching per day, numbers of years teaching, or age. Another study by Smith et al. (17) looked at 554 high school teachers and 220 people not employed in teaching and found that teachers were more likely than controls to define themselves as having a voice problem (36% vs. 1%, $p < 0.05$), having a weak or effortful voice ($p < 0.05$), and having a higher frequency of physical discomfort with speaking ($p < 0.05$). One reason for this finding may be because teaching is such a vocally demanding occupation that even a minor impairment is noted and reported.

There has been relatively little investigation into the environmental and ergonomic risk factors for voice disorders in teachers. Preciado et al. (18) found more prevalent symptoms in females rather than males (19.3% vs. 15.6%), thus confirming previous studies, but also found that teachers in the lowest grades were at increased risk. The numbers of teachers complaining of voice problems were highest in nursery and elementary school, and lowest in junior schools (36.4% vs. 25% vs. 20.8%, respectively). Other factors associated with an increased frequency of vocal disorders were the physical size of the classroom, larger student numbers, longer classroom hours, and higher noise levels.

Despite many authors concluding that the high risk nature of the teaching profession predisposes for occupational voice disorders, Mattiske et al. (19) reviewed published research papers and concluded that the evidence was in fact inconclusive due to the cross-sectional nature of most of the studies and lack of statistical control in their design.

All of the above are significant for the design and prevention of voice disorders in this group and are revisited later.

Singers

Another occupational group that has been highlighted as experiencing a higher prevalence of voice disorders is singers (Fig. 1). Self-reported voice problems in singers have been described in several studies. Miller and Verdolini (20) looked at the frequency of self-reported voice problems in voice or singing teachers by sampling 10% of the membership of the National Association of Teachers of Singing in the United States. Each recipient also received a second questionnaire to be completed by a friend or colleague who was not a singer. One hundred twenty-five singers and 49 controls completed the questionnaires. Twenty-one percent of singing teachers and 18% of controls thought that they currently had a voice problem; however, 64% of teachers and only 33% of controls reported a voice problem in the past. Risk factors for the singing teachers and nonsinging teachers included a history of past voice problems. This increased the risk of a current voice disorder by a factor of five. Current use of specific dehydrating medications increased the risk by three. Female gender and a younger age also increased the risk.

Sapir et al. (15) looked at university voice students and found that, in a questionnaire, 13% were symptom-free, 26% had just one or two symptoms, and 61% had more than three symptoms. Thirty-five (46%) had enough symptoms to seek medical help. Students with multiple symptoms were more likely to be depressed, anxious, frustrated and worried; to miss performances; to forego auditions; and to speak in a voice too low in pitch.

When looking at different types of singers, Perkner et al. (21) compared three specific types of performer—opera, musical theatre, and contemporary (not rock) singers—with

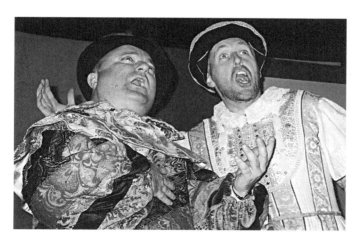

Figure 1 Singers are a recognized group at risk of voice loss due to intense prolonged and repetitive vocal use.

"friendship" controls. They found a significant increase in voice disorders in the singers (44% vs. 21% in "friends") and in voice disability (69% vs. 41% in "friends"), but no difference was found among the different styles of singer.

But how individuals perceive voice problems is important, particularly when research depends on self reports. Kitch and Oates (22) reported that, when vocally fatigued, actors rated the "power" aspects of their voice as most affected whereas singers rated the "dynamic" features as most affected. This emphasizes the importance of considering the different ways the impact of a voice problem affects individuals and the potential to cause different degrees of disability depending on the work task involved.

But it is not just perception of a problem that has been found to be important. White and Verdolini (23) looked at differences in how individuals present at clinics for medical treatment. They looked at gospel singers who were attending voice clinics in the United States and found that African-American singers were more likely than Caucasians to be influenced by what others thought about seeking medical help. In contrast, Caucasian singers sought help if they thought their own voices were affected. This has implications both for research and for interpretation of studies involving hospital clinic attendees, as there appear to be socio-societal and cultural influences on presentation behavior that may introduce bias. The amount of knowledge about the causation of voice disorders may also vary between those who sing for a living—the professional voice users—and those who use their voices at work, and this may influence presentation.

Aerobics Instructors

A number of reports have recently appeared in the literature describing voice problems in aerobics instructors (Fig. 2). The demands of the job require verbal instructions to be given to clients at the same time as performing often strenuous exercise. This makes control of breathing and airflow movement more difficult. Many instructors use microphones (most frequently radio microphones) to reduce the amount of vocal projection necessary in large dance studios, but the acoustics are often such that coordination is still necessary and there can be significant demands placed on young and inexperienced voices.

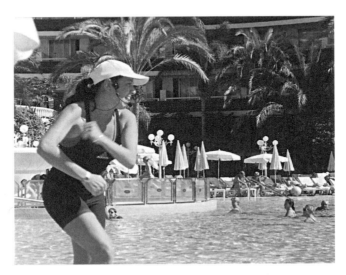

Figure 2 Teaching aqua-aerobics requires intensive voice use and projection combined with physical exercise. Use of a microphone lessens the vocal load.

Long et al. (24) carried out a questionnaire study of 54 aerobics instructors in Alabama. Forty-four percent reported experiencing voice loss and 42.6% reported partial loss during or after instructing a class. Overall, the results showed a significant number of instructors experienced voice loss and episodes of hoarseness. Sore throats unrelated to illness were also increased in the group, related to shouting instruction and cues to clients. The study also identified that very few instructors had any training in vocal hygiene techniques. This study found no effect of microphone use, but the authors commented that the finding may have been due to the availability and access to such equipment and the pre-established habits of the instructors. Previous research on aerobics instructors by Heidel and Torgerson (25) has shown that aerobics instructors experienced an increase in symptomatology in cold weather and this earlier work also confirmed the increased risk for this occupational group.

This occupation, however, needs to be looked at holistically. Work in Japan not only confirmed laryngeal discomfort but also identified leg and calf pain which was significantly related to the number of dance classes per week (26). An ergonomic approach looking at all aspects of repetitive behaviors is thus needed to prevent occupational injury in this group.

Cheerleaders

The vocal behavior of cheerleaders has also been reported as a risk of voice cord pathology (27). Investigations on cheerleaders have indicated that they have a number of characteristics similar to aerobics instructors. These are vocalization while exercising, pyknic or athletic body type, display of "hyperkinetic movements of phonation," and a tendency to develop vocal nodules. Cheerleaders have also been found to suffer from excessive and more frequent hoarseness (28).

Telemarketers

Compared to teachers, relatively little has been published about this occupational group. Jones et al. (29), however, looked at the prevalence of problems in this group and compared it to that in the general population. They also looked at the effects of voice symptoms on productivity. Three hundred and seventy-three employees from six firms were invited to complete a survey. Three hundred and four (81%) responses were compared with those from 187 community college students similar in age, sex, smoking behavior, and educational level. Telemarketers were found to be twice as likely to report one or more symptoms of vocal attrition compared to controls after adjusting for age, sex, and smoking status $(p < 0.001)$. Thirty-one percent of those surveyed reported that their symptoms affected their work. These respondents were more likely to be female $(p < 0.001)$; to smoke $(p < 0.02)$; to take drying medications $(p < 0.001)$; to have sinus problems $(p < 0.04)$; to have frequent colds $(p < 0.001)$ and dry mouth $(p < 0.001)$; and to be sedentary $(p < 0.001)$. The researchers concluded that telemarketers had a higher prevalence of voice problems that affected productivity and the risk factors for these problems were modifiable (Fig. 3).

Teachers, singers, actors, cheerleaders, aerobics inst-ructors, and telemarketers, therefore, figure prominently in published research as groups at risk. The studies, however, are almost always cross-sectional rather than prospective and many are without controls. Other case reports of occupa-tional hoarseness, e.g., in obstetricians (30), have been pub-lished but the literature contains no general data to provide a background prevalence of hoarseness, sore throat, etc. in working and nonworking populations; therefore, any estima-tion of increased prevalence in any one occupational group is not conclusive. The literature has, however, identified important potential biases in studies involving clinic atten-dees, whosepresentation for treatment not only depends on their perception of a voice problem but also on how significant the voice problem affects their ability to do their job. Such a finding means caution is needed in interpreting studies that tend to suggest that a condition is found frequently among an occupational group because that particular occupational group makes up a large portion of attendees at a clinic. It more likely reflects other several other factors, including the diffi-culties those individuals have in performing their usual job.

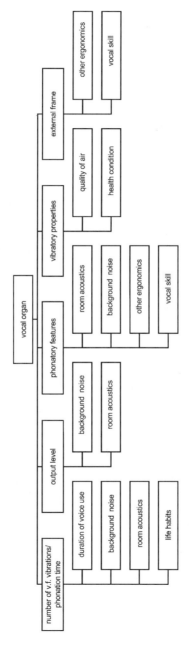

Figure 3 Telemarketers have been found to be at increased risk of voice problems.

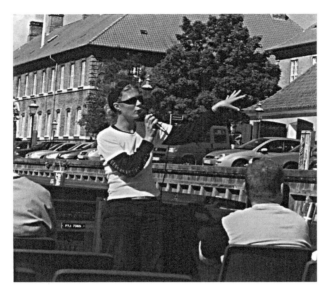

Figure 4   Other groups of workers with essential voice use include tour guides, particularly if working outdoors or in poor acoustic environments.

REFERENCES

1. National Centre for Voice and Speech. Occupational and Voice Data. National Centre Iowa City IA US, 1993.

2. Laukkanen A-M: On speaking voice exercises. PhD thesis. Tampere, University of Tampere, 1995.

3. Ramig LO, Verdolini K. Treatment efficacy; voice disorders. J Speech Lang Hear Res 1998; 41:101–106.

4. Morely DE. A ten-year survey of speech disorders among university students. J Speech Hear Disord 1952:25–31.

5. Laguaite JK. Adult voice screening. J Speech Hear Disord 1972; 37:147–151.

6. Worrall L, Hickson L, Dodd B. Screening for communication impairment in nursing homes and hostels. Aust J Hum Commun Disord 1993; 21:53–64.

7. Coyle SM, Weinrick BD, Semple JC. Shifts in relative prevalence of laryngeal pathology in a treatment seeking population. J Voice 2001; 15:424–440.

8. Verdolini K, Ramig LO. Review: occupational risks for a voice problem. Log Phon Vocol 2001; 26:37–46.

9. Fritzell B. Voice disorders and occupations. Log Phon Vocology 1996; 21:7–12.

10. Titze IR, Lemke J, Montequin D. Populations in the US work force who rely on voice as a primary tool of trade. A preliminary report. J Voice 1997; 11:254–256.

11. Lejska J. Occupational voice disorders in teachers. Pracovini Lekarstvi 1967; 19:119–121.

12. Marks JB. A comparative study of voice problems among teachers and civil service workers. Masters thesis. University of MinnesotaMinneapolis, US1985.

13. Smith E, Gray M, Dove, S, Kirchner L, Heras H. Frequency and effects of teachers voice problems. J Voice 1997; 11:81–87.

14. Russell A, Oates J, Greenwood K. A survey of self-reported voice problems by school teachers in South Australia. 26th Annual Symposium: Care of the Professional Voice, Philadelphia, Pennsylvania, US, 2–7, June 1997.

15. Sapir S, Keidar A, Marthers-Schmidt B. Vocal attrition in teachers : survey findings. Eur J Disord Commun 1993; 4:223–244.

16. Smith E, Kirchner HL, Taylor M, Hoffman H, Lemke JH. Voice problems among teachers: differences in gender and teaching characteristics. J Voice 1998; 12:328–334.

17. Smith E, Lemke J, Taylor M, Kirchner HL, Hoffman H. Frequency of voice problems among teachers and other occupations. J Voice 1998; 12:480–488.

18. Preciado JA, Garcia Tapia R, Infante JC. Prevalence of voice disorders among educational professionals. Factors contributing to their appearance or their persistence. Acta Otorrinolaringology Espania 1998; 49(2):137–142.

19. Mattiske JA, Oates JM, Greenwood KM. Vocal problems among teachers: a review of prevalence, causes, prevention, and treatment. J Voice 1998; 12(4):489–499.

20. Miller M, Verdolini K. Frequency of voice problems reported by teachers of singing and control subjects and risk factors. J Voice 1995; 31:68–69.

21. Perkner JJ, Fennelly KP, Balkisson R, Bucher Bartelsen B, Ruttender J, Wood RP, Phyland DJ, Oates J, Greenwood KM. Self-reported voice problems among three groups of professional singers. J Voice 1999; 13:602–611.

22. Kitch JA, Oates J. The perceptual features of vocal fatigue as self reported in a group of singers and actors. J Voice 1994; 8(3):207–214.

23. White E, Verdolini K. Frequency of voice problems in gospel versus non-gospel choral singers. 24th Annual Symposium: Care of the Professional Voice, Philadelphia, Pennsylvania, US, 5–10, June 1995.

24. Long J, Willford HN, Scharff Olsen M, Wolfe V. Voice problems and risk factors among aerobics instructors. J Voice 1998; 12:197–201.

25. Heidel SE, Torgerson JK. Vocal problems among aerobics instructors and aerobics participants. J Commun Disord 1993; 26(3):179–191.

26. Komura Y, Inaba R, Fujita S, Mirbod SM, Yoshida H, Nagata C, Iwata H. Health condition of female aerobic dance instructors. Subjective symptoms and related factors. Sangyo Igaku 1992: 34:326–334.

27. Reich A, McHenry M, Keaton A. A survey of dysphonic episodes on high-school cheerleaders. Lang Speech Hear Serv Sch 1986; 17:63–71.

28. Reich A, Wilson DK. In: Voice Problems in Children. Baltimore, MD: Williams & Wilkins, 1992.

29. Jones K, Sigmon J, Hock L, Nelson E, Sullivan M, Ogren F. Prevalence and risk factors for voice problems among telemarketers. Arch Otolaryngol Head Neck Surg 2002; 128(5): 571–577.

30. Dowailby JM. The hoarse obstetrician. Arch Otolaryngol Head Neck Surg 1992; 118(3):343–344.

3

The Etiology of Voice Disorders

COMMON PATHOLOGICAL CONDITIONS
THAT CAUSE VOICE DISORDERS

The most common pathologies of the voice are described here. A large majority of disorders are related to abuse, misuse, and psychogenic factors (1–9). This is particularly true in the context of occupational voice disorders. Major consideration should also be given to chemical and environmental issues. In a clinical environment, all voice problems are considered as a potential consequence of serious medical diseases (including laryngeal carcinoma) until proven otherwise. For this reason, this chapter begins with an overview of diseases and medical conditions that commonly affect the voice.

Diseases and Medical Conditions that Commonly Affect the Voice

Neurological Voice Disorders

Central or peripheral nervous system lesions can result in a voice disorder. Typical voice quality characteristics are identifiable in different nervous system disorders (2). A change in voice quality may be one of the first signs of an early stage progressive neurological disorder (e.g., myasthenia gravis, parkinsonism, motor neurone disease/amyotrophoic lateral sclerosis) (2). However, more commonly, the voice disorder presents a part of a complex oral, pharyngeal, and laryngeal disorder resulting from paralysis and paresis of multiple organs of voice, speech, and swallowing (10).

Systemic Disease

The association between autoimmune diseases and voice disorders has been well documented—for example, as seen in laryngeal rheumatoid arthritis (11), systemic lupus erythematosus (12), and Sjogren's syndrome (13). Systemic infection (e.g., tuberculosis, syphilitic inflammation) may also have voice change manifestations (12). These conditions are obviously rare in the general population, but voice complications seem high in individuals with these diseases and infections.

Endocrinological Disorders

Endocrine-related (insufficient androgen secretion) voice problems in males are rare, and should not be confused with mutational falsetto (puberphonia), which is a failure of the male voice to "break" into the adult range in the absence of any other endocrinological disease (14). Some voice changes in females can be related to menstruation (15), pregnancy (16), or menopause (17). This is principally because of the hormonal changes that result in the vocal folds becoming edematous (swollen) and congested. However, other physical and emotional changes that occur simultaneously are also relevant (see Ref. 2 for a full review). Thyroid gland dysfunction (both hypo- and hyperthyroidism) is well known to be related to voice changes, particularly in women (18,19).

Benign Neoplasms

There are a number of benign growths that may occur on the vibrating edge of the vocal folds or in the surrounding structures of the larynx. Most of these lesions require stroboscopy (see Chapter 4) for accurate examination and assessment of their specific effect on the mechanics of voicing. These neoplasms include viral papilloma (20), laryngeal mucous gland retention cysts, epidermoid cysts (3), and vocal process granulomas (4). Vocal nodules are also a type of benign growth but are caused by vocal misuse and abuse. (The reasons are discussed in a relevant section later). Malignant growths are rare, and hence the diagnosis and treatment of these lesions are not discussed in this book.

Respiratory Conditions

Normal voice requires a constant and controlled expiratory flow of air through the vocal folds to generate a regular vibration of the vocal folds. Hence, inspiratory and expiratory respiration problems can adversely affect the voice. Reduced respiratory efficiency affects not only the quality of the vocal sound but also phrase length, speech rate, and breathing patterns for conversational or prolonged speech. Common respiratory conditions that affect voice include asthma, bronchitis, emphysema, and chronic obstructive airways (9) disease. Furthermore, many studies have shown that common medical treatments for these conditions (e.g., inhaled corticosteroids) further exacerbate the dysphonia because of mucosal irritation and drying (13,21,22).

Voice Disorders Caused by Voice Misuse

A large majority of voice disorders are because of individual vocal abuse and misuse.* Recent analyses of voice clinic attendance

---

*In this text, the terms vocal "abuse" and vocal "misuse" are used interchangeably. Previous authors have tried to distinguish between these concepts with little success and minimal value.

and diagnosis provide clear evidence to support this (1–3,23). Voice abuse and misuse refers to the way an individual's voice is used and cared for (or not). Occupational voice users are at high risk of disorders of this nature. This is mainly because of the type of voice use (e.g., aggressive or forceful voice quality, loud voice, talking over background noise, loud singing), the workplace environment (e.g., dusty, dry, smoky), and the consequences of not being able to fully use his/her voice for the job. Rarely is the occupational voice risk based upon the amount of voice use alone (after all, there are many teachers, telemarketers, lawyers, singers, etc., who do not have voice problems). The concept of recovery rate may be important here—prolonged and excessive physical activity requires sufficient time to recover.

However, occupational voice demands are not the only risk factor in abuse/misuse-related voice disorders. Gender is important because female voices are higher pitched; hence the vocal folds vibrate at a greater frequency. The "frequency of collision" of the vocal folds may be implicated in the development of dysphonia (24). Other studies have suggested that genetically determined differences in the membranous portions of the vocal folds may mean that some individuals have more "robust" voices than others (25,26). In addition, the risks of developing a disorder are further heightened in the context of concomitant health issues—either a temporary condition (e.g., laryngitis, chronic cough) or a more permanent problem (e.g., poor respiratory function). These are discussed further later.

One of the main roles of the voice pathologist (a speech-and-language therapist who specializes in voice disorders) is to determine the presence and nature of relevant vocally abusive components (23). These components are often interactive and include habitual voicing patterns, posture and breathing patterns, laryngeal irritants, work environment issues, compensatory voicing behaviors, and psychological issues. Each of these is studied in detail below.

Habitual Voicing Patterns

If a speaker constantly uses his/her voice with excessive laryngeal tension, force, and constriction, then a voice disorder is likely to occur. Many voice disorder textbooks refer to this strained pattern of voicing as "hyperfunctional" (4,6) or muscle tension dysphonia (8). Oates (27) lists a common set of vocally abusive voicing patterns which include:

- Speaking (or singing) with excessive loudness
- Speaking (or singing) with excessive high or low pitch levels
- Yelling or screaming
- Speaking (or singing) with excessive laryngeal muscle tension
- Forced, strained, or effortful speech or singing
- Excessive coughing and throat clearing
- Phonation during effortful closure of the larynx (e.g., during weightlifting)

Posture and Breathing Patterns

Many authors identify postural misalignment (especially of the head and neck) as a common cause of muscle tension in the larynx (2,3,5,6,8). The assumption is that the muscle tone in the vocal tract and larynx will be adversely affected by muscle tension in surrounding and related structures. Oates (27) identifies a number of general postural misalignments that may result in concomitant voice problems. These include:

- Hyperextension or hyperflexion of the neck and mandible
- "Slumping" of the spine
- Raising of the shoulders
- Exaggerated position of the pelvis

Lieberman (28) adds several other key observations, including spinal asymmetry and torso rotation, both of which appear to pull the larynx away from the midline. He also advocates structured observation of head position. This, of course, should take into account "habitual" position at work as well as elsewhere. The interested reader is referred to Lieberman's accounts (28) and observations for further information.

Perhaps more obviously, restricted mobility of the muscle structures of or around the vocal tract may result in vocal hyperfunction. A number of standard textbooks (2,3,5,6,8) describe these features, which include:

- Temporomandibular joint tension (i.e., jaw clenching)
- Excessive tension in the base of tongue muscles
- Excessive tongue retraction
- Tongue body hypertonicity (e.g., at rest, tongue pushed against back of lower teeth)
- Laryngeal tenderness when touched/manipulated
- High position of the larynx during phonation

Lieberman (28) describes a full assessment protocol for these features. Clearly, if any of these postural features are prevalent during times of prolonged talking (e.g., "shoulder cradling" the telephone, screen position for call center workers, chair–desk positioning), then the potential for voice problems is even greater.

Finally, inappropriate and inefficient breathing patterns may lead to vocally abusive and hyperfunctional voice problems. Clearly, poor posture may restrict the diaphragm and result in poor control of air for speech (5). This often results in inefficient air use, which most commonly manifests itself as a complaint of not being able to complete phrases in one breath or running out of air toward the end of a sentence. Other habitual breathing anomalies include excessive air bursts at the start of sentences (a common feature among teachers) and talking in excessively low or high airflow rates (characteristic among aerobic instructors). Insufficient and/or inappropriate breath control for voicing is likely to result in laryngeal overcompensation and subsequent muscle tension (2,3,5,6,8).

Laryngeal Irritants

A large majority of the substances that are known to irritate the larynx are either inhaled (airborne) or are dehydrants. Some of these are listed in Table 1.

Although it is not clear why some voices appear to be more irritated by these agents than others, the effects are common. Oates (27) reports that the general effect of these

Table 1 Common Laryngeal Irritants

Airborne/inhaled substances	Dehydrating substances
Tobacco/marijuana smoke	Alcohol
Chemical fumes	Caffeine
Dust	Recreational drugs (oral)
Excessive dry air	Oral medications including
Air pollutants	antihistamines, decongestants,
Allergens	cough suppressants,
Inhaled corticosteroids	antidepressants, and
	antihypertensive agents (3,5)

irritants may be increased viscosity of laryngeal lubrication (thickened and sticky secretions) and drying of vocal fold mucosa. These laryngeal irritations frequently lead to increased laryngeal strain on phonation, as well as throat clearing and coughing. Such responses only serve as additional abusive habits that further damage the vibrating edge of the vocal folds.

Morrison et al. (29) describe a constellation of symptoms that may be termed as "irritable larynx syndrome." They suggest that this hypersensitivity of the laryngeal structures is caused by neuronal changes in the CNS. They postulate that in these patients, the larynx is "hyper-excitable" and that it reacts disproportionately to sensory stimulation (e.g., dust, perfumes, chemical smells, smoke, spicy foods). In almost all cases, these patients will have a concomitant voice problem.

Finally, it is now commonly agreed that gastro oesophageal reflux (peptic acid reflux from the stomach) is a major cause of laryngeal irritation. Koufman (30) suggests that as much as 70% of voice patients may have this disease. If the refluxed acid reaches the larynx, the mucosa is subject to surface tissue irritation and subsequent voice changes. Distinguishing symptoms may include regular "heartburn," regurgitation, or dyspepsia (painful swallowing and digestion) (2). However, importantly, recent studies suggest that less than 50% of voice patients with clinically significant reflux report these classic overt symptoms (31).

Poor Vocal Knowledge/Skill

Poor vocal technique will result in less efficient and effective voice production, which is more susceptible to strain and misuse. The appropriate combination of the use of air flow and vocal fold tension produces a remarkably resilient vibratory mechanism, which is capable of many thousands of vibrations a day (see Chapter 2). Similar to any muscle activity, inefficient and poorly coordinated movement will result in muscle strain and fatigue. Furthermore, a lack of knowledge of voice care will additionally compromise the health of the structures and will result in further deterioration in performance. For example, repeated throat clearing, speaking at an inappropriate pitch, and singing outside of the comfortable range will all contribute to an excessive demand on the voice, which will eventually result in deterioration.

Work Environment

The next chapter is devoted to the careful consideration of the work environment and its potential contribution to occupational voice disorders. Clearly, seating and desk positioning (for postural strain), ambient/background noise levels (for continual voice projection), and air quality (for inhaled laryngeal irritants) are all highly relevant. The amount of talking and at what volume levels are also an important consideration, and these issues are discussed in a later chapter.

Compensatory Voicing Behaviors

A number of medical conditions can result in inflammation and irritation of the vocal fold mucosa. These include viral or bacterial laryngeal infections, allergic reactions, and chronic sinusitis (5). Furthermore, diseases of the respiratory system (e.g., asthma, chronic obstructive airways disease) limit breath support for adequate speech. As described above, the vocal fold mucosa is also vulnerable to a large number of laryngeal irritants. In addition to the direct effect these conditions have on the voice, it is likely that the speaker may develop further compensatory behaviors that may worsen the voice problems. Oates (27), for example, describes a case of infective laryngitis where the vocal folds have become inflamed and swollen. The speaker is likely to clear his/her throat or cough in an attempt to alleviate the irritation or to speak with increased muscle effort to produce stronger voice. Both compensatory behaviors are likely to increase voice problems and encourage the "habitualization" of vocal abuse and misuse characteristics.

Chronic sinusitis with purulent discharge will similarly irritate the vocal fold mucosa with the same outcome being likely. Colton and Casper (6) describe patients with compromised airway conditions and the consequential voice abuse (coughing, clearing throat) and voice misuse (vocal strain and forcing) features that frequently occur. This concept of inappropriate and increasingly damaging compensatory vocal behaviors is central to the understanding of how and why a voice problem may be prolonged or be perpetuated beyond the initial dysphonic episode. Furthermore, it helps explain the slow onset of many voice abuse/misuse disorders as the patient gradually adopts further compensatory behaviors in a misguided attempt to overcome voice difficulties.

Psychological Issues

Mathieson (2) points out that there is a strong link between voice abuse/misuse and a speaker's personality and emotional status. This helps explain why a voice-disordered person may describe severe levels of personal disability and distress (32,33). A whole range of human emotions can be reflected in the human voice (34–39). Extreme and persistent states of heightened emotion are therefore likely to involve vocal strain and high vocal demand. Personal stress and anxiety may somatize into muscle tension, and the voice musculature would appear to be particularly vulnerable. Ironically for such people, their voice is least functionally useful at a time when they might need it most. Oates (27) describes a number of common psychogenic features that result in increased levels of intrinsic and extrinsic laryngeal muscle tension

Table 2 Commonly Reported Psychological Features Associated with Voice Misuse and Abuse

Personality characteristics	Chronic life stresses	Emotional events
Aggressiveness	Anger	Relationship breakdown
Poor stress coping skills	Hostility	Work stress
Loud, extrovert	Pain (emotional and physical)	Hectic, out-of-control lifestyle
Forceful and dominant	Resentment	Self and family illness

and forced phonation. These characteristics are listed in Table 2.

Clinical Signs of Voice Misuse

The complex set of contributory factors described above illustrates the difficulty in the differential diagnosis of voice abuse and misuse. A detailed case history may reveal a number of issues pertaining to laryngeal irritants, work environment, levels of vocal hygiene, and psychosocial factors. Structured and detailed observation of posture and breathing is a routine part of all specialist speech-and-voice pathologists (speech-and-language therapists who specialize in voice disorders). Perceptual auditory assessment is likely to reveal a strained, forced, breathy, or rough voice quality. "Hard glottal attack" may also be present—this refers to a perceptual quality of forced onset of voicing. Other voice laboratory assessments may include measurements of sound pressure levels, speaking pitch (habitual and total range), vocal fold vibratory patterns, and airflow during phonation (40). Video-laryngeal-endoscopy is essential to exclude other diseases (as described at the beginning of this chapter). Pathological changes may occur on the vibrating edge of the vocal folds as a result of repeated collision trauma of forced and strained voicing (3–5). These lesions (e.g., nodules or polyps) commonly occur at the center of the membranous portion of the vocal folds—the place where the mechanical impact of vocal folds vibration is greatest (2,3). However, not all cases of vocal hyperfunction result in pathological changes in the larynx. Morrison and Rammage (8) describe a series of laryngeal configurations that are indicative of muscle tension dysphonia. All of these reveal excessive muscle effort and inappropriate recruitment of alternative or surrounding muscle structures. Endoscopic (and stroboscopic) examination may also reveal clinical signs of gastroesophageal reflux (30), mucosal dehydration, sites of minor laryngeal trauma, and/ or limited muscle elasticity with different voicing tasks (3).

In conclusion, voice problems can be caused by a wide variety of medical, behavioral, and psychogenic causes. Differential diagnosis is frequently complex and requires multiprofessional collaboration. Occupational voice disorders are most likely to be caused by features of voice abuse and misuse. These aspects often interact and result in a spiralling cycle of symptoms. However, diagnosis of a voice abuse/misuse problem can only be done following the elimination of other diseases and medical conditions that may cause dysphonia. Additional diagnostic complications arise when relevant medical conditions are present simultaneously with elements of voice abuse/misuse.

OCCUPATIONAL IRRITANTS AND ENVIRONMENTAL CONDITIONS

The previous section dealt with voice disorders related to misuse and overuse. In this section, we consider some of the occupational and environmental agents that have been reported to affect the voice.

Occupational/Chemical Agents

Perkner et al. (41) reported vocal cord dysfunction because of occupational and environmental irritants in 11 individuals. They conducted a case control study to determine whether the irritant-exposed vocal cord dysfunction group differed from the nonexposed patients. Age matching was carried out. The researchers reported that in the exposed group, chest discomfort and ethnicity were statistically different from the controls but there were no differences between gender, tobacco, smoking habits, or pulmonary function results.

Tanturri et al. (42) described a case of exposure to freon gas, a halogenated hydrocarbon used in refrigeration. Exposure of a worker resulted in the gradual onset of edematous pharyngolaryngitis with multiple symptoms, including pain and difficulty in swallowing, dysphonia, and inspiratory breathlessness.

Roto and Sala (43) described a case of occupational laryngitis attributed to exposure to formaldehyde in a single case report. A nonsmoking dairy foreman was exposed to the chemical for 9 years. Formaldehyde is a sterilizing agent widely used in industry and also used as a preservative. The exposure was from emissions from a milk-packing machine below his office; hence, he was not directly working with the agent. Levels of formaldehyde in air were measured and were found to be 0.03 mg/m^3, a low concentration. The patient complained of prolonged hoarseness and chest tightness, with symptoms developing immediately after entering his office. He began to develop episodes of aphonia in conjunction with pharyngeal irritation. Characteristic of an occupationally related condition, all of the symptoms disappeared when he was on sick leave. He was initially diagnosed as having psychogenic dysphonia, but reacted positively to formaldehyde in a laryngeal provocation test. Hoarseness, reddening of the laryngeal mucosa, and redness and swelling of the vocal cords were all found to have increased after the provocation test, and the abnormalities were still observed 8 hours later. The symptoms subsided 24 hours after the test. In comparison, five healthy control subjects had no reaction to 1 ppm formaldehyde. In this case, the outcome was that the patient was retired on grounds of ill health because of the seriousness of his laryngitis. Unfortunately, the condition continued to deteriorate in 3 years of follow-up during which time he began to react strongly to tobacco smoke and other formaldehyde-containing air impurities. The authors emphasized the importance of occupational history and the use of provocation testing in the diagnostic process. Such accuracy as to the cause of the symptoms can help patients avoid agents likely to exacerbate their condition.

Brown (44) studied a case of dysphonia, dysphagia, and excessive salivary secretions in a rare fatal case of chronic mercury poisoning. The subject was a farmer who used organic mercury as a pesticide and dusted it on oat seeds.

Sechi et al. (45) described acute and persistent parkinsonism, including dysphonia in a 72-year-old Italian male farmer exposed to diquat, another pesticide. They reported that he had been exposed to 10% aqueous diquat dibromide 3 months previously and that 10 minutes after the exposure, he developed reddening of the skin with subsequent hyperkeratosis (localized skin thickening) and reddening (known as injection) of the conjunctiva of the eyes. Other eye symptoms included widespread reddening and excessive tears. The symptoms of irritation resolved after 4 days, but 10 days later he developed severe akathisia (a movement disorder involving shaking). Five days later he became dysphonic. Because of the pattern of onset of the symptoms, the dysphonia was attributed to the chemical exposure rather than to parkinsonism.

The risks of occupational exposure to sulfuric acid, such as might occur in workers involved in battery manufacture, have also been recognized by the National Institute of Occupational Safety and Health (NIOSH), a government body in the United States. They report that the acid is a risk factor for carcinoma of both the larynx and laryngitis (46). Turner (47) also described a case of occupational rhinitis, laryngitis, and dysphonia in a 46-year-old man who worked in shoe manufacturing and had long-term exposure to solvents, including a modified isocyanates-containing product. Methylene chloride (also known as dichloromethane) was also used for cleaning tanks out. The patient saw four ENT surgeons before an occupational history was taken and had sinus washouts that failed to improve his symptoms.

Finally, a review paper by Sala et al. (48) listed agents such as flour, plants, and acid anhydrides (formaldehyde, acrylate compounds, and chemicals used in hairdressing) as potential causes of occupational laryngitis.

Environmental Conditions

Research has suggested links between environmental noise, relative humidity and temperature of inhaled air, and dust as affecting voice production.

Rontal et al. (49) reported a definite association between vocal cord dysfunction and work in noisy environments with incidence levels of 8% (for vocal cord nodules, vocal cord polyps, and chronic laryngitis) in individuals working in high noise environments. In addition to an increased incidence of vocal pathology, they also reported that workers in noisy environments had a 30% incidence rate for recurrent vocal cord dysfunction following surgery. Females were found to be at more risk than males. Other researchers have also documented the link between work in a noisy environment and dysphonia (50), but not all studies have found associations between hoarseness and noise exposure (51).

Smoky and dusty atmospheres have also been implicated in occupational voice disorders primarily in the theater and opera. Richter et al. (52) found levels of dust and low humidity outside the range recommended by the German government for the generic workplace. They also found high temperatures and showed that by installing humidification units and cleaning, levels of dust and dryness and temperature of the air reduced.

Dry atmospheres were also identified by Hemler et al. (53) and Vintturi et al. (54) as leading to vocal dysfunction. Hemler used sheep larynges to show that dry dehydrating air of relative humidity 0% produced more stiffness and viscous cover of the folds than humidified (100%) air ($p < 0.001$). Ventura and colleagues looked at central fatigue, neck/shoulder/back symptoms, dryness of the throat and mouth, throat and voice symptoms in both men and women exposed to eight combinations of high (>65%) or low (< 65%) humidity, and high [> 65 dB (SPL)] and low [< 65 dB (SPL)] speech levels in sitting or standing positions. They found statistically significant differences for central fatigue (humidity had clear effects) and symptoms of neck/shoulder/back discomfort (gender, posture, and humidity had effects, more so in females than males).

Low humidity produced more symptoms than high humidity and standing, more symptoms than the seated position. In a different study, Vintturi et al. (55) showed that low humidity led to more hyperfunction of the voice, while researchers in the Netherlands have shown how the human voice is very sensitive to even short periods of inhaled air of low humidity (56).

It is not just the humidity and moisture content of inhaled air that is important. Individuals who breathe through their mouths (perhaps trying to avoid noxious smells in the workplace) have been shown to have superficial drying of the vocal fold mucosa (57). One double blind placebo-controlled study looking at hydration found that there were improvements in voice and laryngeal appearance in individuals with nodules or polyps after 5 days of hydration compared to 5 consecutive days of placebo treatment. It is difficult to generalize the normal worker from such a clinical study, but it does suggest that hydration is an important factor in maintaining vocal health.

The published literature contains relatively few controlled studies of occupational voice disorders arising from workplace exposure to irritants or environmental conditions. Most of the literature relates to case reports.

However, the impact of a permanent voice disorder in workers can have a profound effect on an individual's occupational and social functioning. In investigating possible occupational causes of voice disorders, it is important that details are taken of chemicals to which workers may be exposed and of the working conditions so that investigation is focused and further ill-health can be prevented by management of exposure.

REFERENCES

1. Carding PN. Voice pathology in the United Kingdom. BMJ 2003; 327:514–515.

2. Mathieson L. Greene and Mathieson's The Voice and its Disorders. 6th ed. London: Whurr, 2001.

3. Harris T, Harris S, et al. The Voice Clinic Handbook. London: Whurr, 2000.

4. Dworkin JP, Meleca RJ. Vocal Pathologies: Diagnosis, Treatment, and Case Studies. San Diego: Singular, 1997.

5. Freeman M, Fawcus M. Voice Disorders and their Management. Whurr, 2000.

6. Colton RH, Casper JK. Understanding Voice Problems: A Physiological Perspective for Diagnosis and Treatment. 2nd ed. Baltimore, MD: Williams and Wilkins, 1996.

7. Gleeson M ed. Scott and Brown's Otolaryngology and Head and Neck Surgery. 10th ed. London: Arnold. In press.

8. Morrison M, Rammage L. The Management of Voice Disorders. London: Chapman and Hall Medical, 1994.

9. Carding PN, Wade A. Managing dysphonia caused by misuse and overuse. BMJ 2000; 276:1544–1545.

10. McNeil MR, Rosenbeck JC, Aronson AE. The Dysartrias: Physiology, Acoustics, Perception, and Management. San Diego, California: College-Hill Press, 1984.

11. Jurik AG, Pederson U, Norgard A. Rheumatoid arthritis of the crico-aryntenoid joints: a case of laryngeal obstruction due to acute and chronic joint changes. Laryngoscope 1985; 95:846.

12. Teitel AD, MacKenzie CR, Stern R, Paget SA. Laryngeal involvement in systemic lupus erythematosus. Sem Arthritis Rheum 1992; 22:203–214.

13. Clarke PM, Durham SR, Perry A, MacKay IS. Objective measurement of voice change caused by inhaled steroids. Voice 1992; 1:63–66.

14. Livesey J, Carding PN. Puberphonia or the male voice that will not break. Aust Voice 1996; 8:34–38.

15. Abitol J, de Brux J, Millot G, et al. Does a hormonal vocal cord cycle exist in women? Study of vocal pre-menstrual syndrome in voice performers by videostroboscopy–glottography and cytology on 38 women. J Voice 1989; 3:157–162.

16. Flach M, Schwickardi H, Simon R. What influence do menstruation and pregnancy have on a trained singing voice? Folia Phoniatrica 1969; 21:199–200.

17. Sataloff RT. Professional Voice: The Science and Art of Clinical Care. New York: Raven Press, 1991.

18. Ritter FN. The effects of hyperthyroidism upon the ear, nose, and throat. Laryngoscope 1967; 77:1427–1428.

19. Allen GW. Neoplasms of the thyroid gland. In: English GM, ed. Otolaryngology. New York: Harper and Row, 1984.

20. Bone RC, Feren AP, Nahum AM. Laryngeal papillomatosis: immunologic and viral basis for therapy. Laryngoscope 1976; 86:341–346.

21. Goldberg J, Kovarsky J. Beclomethasone dipropriate inhalation treatment for chronic hoarseness in rheumatic diseases. Arthritis Rheumatol 1983; 26:1412–1415.

22. Watkin K, Ewanowski S. Effects of aerosol corticosteroids on the voice; triamcinolone, acetonide, and beclomethasone diproionate. J Speech Hear Res 1985; 28:301–305.

23. Koschkee DL, Rammage L. Voice Care in the Medical Setting. San Diego, London: Singular Publishing Group, 1997.

24. Titze I. Biomechanics and distributed mass models of vocal fold vibration. In: Stevens KN, Hirano M, eds. Vocal Fold Physiology. Tokyo: University of Tokyo Press, 1981.

25. Gray SD, Hirano M, Sato K. Molecular and cellular structure of vocal fold tissue. In: Titze IR, ed. Vocal Fold Physiology: Frontiers of Basic Science. San Diego, California: Singular Publishing Group, 1993.

26. Child DR, Johnson TS. Preventable and non-preventable causes of voice disorders. Sem Speech Lang 1991; 12:1–13.

27. Oates J. Chapter 7. In: Freeman M, Fawcus M, eds. Voice Disorders and their Management. London: Whurr, 2000.

28. Lieberman J. Chapter 6. In: Harris T, Harris S, et al., eds. The Voice Clinic Handbook. London: Whurr, 2000.

29. Morrison M, Rammage L, Emami AJ. The irritable larynx syndrome. J Voice 1999; 13:447–455.

30. Koufman J. Reflux and voice disorders. In: Rubin J, et al., eds. Diagnosis and Treatment of Voice Disorders. New York: Igaku-Shoin, 1995.

31. Forrest LA, Weed H. *Candida laryngitis* appearing as leuko-plakia and GERD. J Voice 1998; 12:91–95.

32. Ramig LO, Verdolini K. Treatment efficacy: voice disorders. J Speech Lang Hear Res 1998; 41:S101–S166.

33. Wilson JA, Deary IJ, Millar A, MacKenzie K. The quality of life impact of dysphonia. Clin Otolaryngol. In press.

34. Ryan EB, Giles H, Sebastian RJ. An integrative perspective for the study of attitudes towards language variation. In: Ryan EB, Giles H, eds. The Social Psychology of Language. London: Edward Arnold, 1982.

35. Scherer K. Expression of emotion in voice and music. J Voice 1995; 9:235–248.

36. Moses PJ. The Voice of Neurosis. New York: Grune and Stratton, 1954.

37. White A, Deary IJ, Wilson JA. Psychiatric disturbance and personality traits in dysphonic patients. Eur J Disord Commun 1997; 32:307–314.

38. Gudykunst WB. Intergroup communication. In: Giles H. ed. The Social Psychology of Language and Communication Studies. London: Edward Arnold, 1986.

39. Scherer K, Giles H. Social Markers in Speech. Cambridge: Cambridge University Press, 1979.

40. Baken RJ, Orlikoff RE. Clinical Measurement of Speech and Voice. 2nd ed. San Diego: Singular, 2000.

41. Perkner JJ, Fennelly KP, Balkissoon R, Bartelsen B, Ruttenber AJ, Wood RP II, Newman LS. Irritant associated vocal cord dysfunction. J Occup Environ Med 1998; 40:136–143.

42. Tanturri G, Pia F, Benzi-M. A case of oedematous pharyngo-laryngitis in a subject occupationally exposed to freon gas. Med del Lavoro 1988; 79:219–222.

43. Roto P, Sala E. Occupational laryngitis caused by formalde-hyde: A case report. Am J Ind Med 1996; 29:275–277.

44. Brown IA. Chronic mercurialism. Arch Neurol Psychiatry 1954; 72:674–681.

45. Sechi GP, Agnetti V, Piredda M, Canu M, Deserra F, Omar HA, Rosati G. Acute and persistent parkinsonism after use of diquat. Neurology 1992; 42:261–262.

46. National Institutes for Occupational Safety and Health. Laryngeal cancer incidence among workers exposed to acid mists. Cancer Causes Control 1997; 8(1):34–38.

47. Turner WE. Chronic rhinitis/laryngitis. N Z Med J 1991; 104:170.

48. Sala E, Hytonen M, Tupasela O, Estlander T. Occupational laryngitis with immediate allergic or immediate type specific chemical hypersensitivity. Clin Otolaryngol 1996; 21(1):42–48.

49. Rontal E, Rontal M, Jacob HJ, Rolnick MI. Vocal cord dysfunction—an industrial health hazard. Ann Otol Rhinol Laryngol 1979; 88:818–821.

50. Otto B, Klajman S, Koldej E, Otto-Sternal W. An analysis of the relation between dysphonia in shipyard workers and working in noise. Bull Inst Marit Trop Med Gydnia 1980; 31 (3–4):185–192.

51. van Dijk FJ, Souman AM, de Vries FF. Non-auditory effects of noise in industry. VI. A final field study in industry. Int Arch Occup Environ Health 1987; 59(2):133–145.

52. Richter B, Lohle E, Maier W, Kliemann B, Verdolini K. Working conditions on stage: climatic considerations. Logoped Phoniatr Vocol 2000; 25(2):80–86.

53. Hemler RJ, Wieneke GH, Lebacq J, Dejonckere PH. Laryngeal mucosa elasticity and viscosity in high and low relative air humidity. Eur Arch Otorhinolaryngol 2001; 258(3): 125–129.

54. Vintturi J, Alku P, Sala E, Sihvo M, Vilkman E. Loading related subjective symptoms during a vocal loading with special reference to gender and some ergonomic factors. Folia Phoniatr Logop 2003; 55(2):55–69.

55. Vintturi J, Alku P, Lauri ER, Sala E, Sihvo M, Vilkman E. Objective analysis of vocal warm up with special reference to ergonomic factors. J Voice 2001; 15(1):36–53.

56. Hemler RJ, Wieneke GH, Dejonckere PH. The effect of relative humidity of inhaled air on acoustic parameters of voice in normal subjects. J Voice 1997; 11(3):295–300.

57. Verdolini-Marston K, Sandage M, Titze IR. Effect of hydration on laryngeal nodules and polyp related and related voice measures. J Voice 1994; 8(1):30–47.

4

Assessment and Diagnosis

This chapter outlines how voice disorders can be assessed in clinical and occupational settings.

CLINICAL DIFFERENTIAL DIAGNOSIS

The clinical differential diagnosis of voice disorders is a complex process that is likely to require the combined expertise of a number of related disciplines (1–8). A change in voice quality (e.g., hoarseness, change in pitch, change in resonance) or vocal performance (e.g., inability to shout, loss of singing voice, inability to talk for long periods of time) may be caused by a variety of pathologies and exacerbated by a

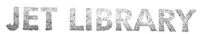

number of additional factors. For these reasons, accurate differential diagnosis is vital, and this process is described in detail below. A comprehensive explanation of all the possible causes of voice disorders lies outside the scope of this work. Whole books have been devoted to this subject, and the interested reader is directed to several classics in the field (2–8).

The Diagnostic Process

Accurate differential diagnosis of a voice disorder requires comprehensive assessment by a specialist voice clinic team. This team primarily consists of a laryngologist and a voice pathologist (a speech therapist/pathologist who specializes in voice disorders) and may also involve other professionals (e.g., psychologist, neurologist, endocrinologist, osteopath) as appropriate (1–8). Assessment should always include a detailed case history, perceptual evaluation of voice quality (listening to how the voice sounds), and laryngeal endoscopie and stroboscopie visualization of the vocal tract during phonation (voicing).

A detailed case history can help identify possible "precipitating, predisposing, and perpetuating factors" (8) that may help explain the voice disorder. Martin (5) states that some professional voice users may have a very intimate and acute knowledge of their voice problems. This may include a good awareness of how and when their voice quality changed; they may even have insight into possible causative factors. The patient's perception of his/her voice problem may provide the skilled clinician with many important clues to help differential diagnosis. Valuable diagnostic features include the pattern of onset, the length of time since onset, and how consistent the dysphonic episodes appear. Case history information should also include information on the amount of voice use the patient routinely has (both at work and outside), the environment in which voice use takes place, the amount of voice training the patient has received in the past, and how the patient has tried to manage the voice problem. It is also important to ascertain how much work time has been lost as a consequence of the voice disorder and whether performance of the usual work duties is currently possible.

The detailed case history can also help identify emotional, psychosocial, and life stresses that may have an impact on the patient's voice. Often patients do not associate these factors with their voice problem and may not, therefore, readily volunteer this information. Patient self-report measures of voice-related quality of life (9–11) can provide further insight into the voice problem from the speaker's perspective. It is important to acknowledge that the impact of a voice problem may be considerable in those who need their voice in order to perform their job. Voice professionals and voice performers may demonstrate high vocal handicap/disability/ distress scores but minimal other "clinical" signs (10,11).

Auditory perceptual evaluation of how the voice sounds can provide essential information to aid differential diagnosis: different vocal characteristics are indicative of different vocal pathologies (2). Speech and language therapists who specialize in voice disorders are highly skilled in perceptual evaluation of voice quality. Features such as instability, hoarseness, low habitual pitch, strain, and breathiness (to name just a few) help the clinician form a hypothesis as to possible laryngeal features that may present on endoscopy.

Endoscopic visualization of the vocal folds and the whole vocal tract is essential for accurate diagnosis (Fig. 1) (3). Endoscopic evaluation of "free" or connected speech can provide important information about behavioral vocal production patterns (12). This may involve endoscopic observation of the patient speaking in a manner similar to that during work (e.g., talking in the classroom, talking above background noise, singing).

Stroboscopic examination (a technique that creates the visual illusion of "slowing down" of vocal fold vibration during phonation) is crucial to exclude subtle laryngeal pathology on the vibrating edges of the vocal folds (3).

More detailed voice testing may include voice "stressing" or vocal loading tasks (for examples, see Ref. 13). These require the patient to perform increasingly demanding vocal tasks (e.g., speaking with a loud voice for a specific amount

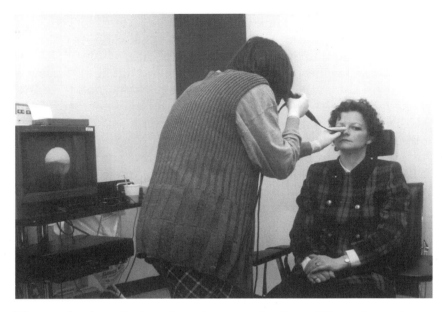

Figure 1 A patient undergoing examination of the voice using a transnasal flexible fibreoptic endoscope. Courtesy of Paul Carding.

of time). A variety of measurements of voice characteristics and performance indices can then be made (e.g., Ref. 13). Clearly, the aim of these procedures is to simulate how the voice functions in a work environment or following excessive vocal demand. These tests have been designed to overcome the common problem of assessing patients who complain of vocal attrition and deterioration with increased use (a common feature of voice abuse and misuse) but who do not present in the clinic with this degree of problem.

Advanced voice clinic services may also use additional diagnostic voice measurement techniques, including electromyography, sound wave analysis of the voice signal, and aerodynamic measurements (9,14). These serve to examine specific characteristics of the vocal mechanism and, in some cases, can be used to instrumentally document aspects of vocal function and change over time (14). Typical features that are measured include the habitual pitch of the voice, the pitch range, habitual vocal loudness, and the regularity of the vocal fold vibration pattern during phonation (9,14).

Multiprofessional discussion of the results of these assessments culminates in a comprehensive differential diagnosis that enables appropriate treatment to commence immediately (3). This process can often be complex and multi-factorial. It is not always immediately obvious which present-ing features are central to the patient's problem and which are peripheral, or which are causative and which are compen-satory. Many diagnostic teams opt for a treatment program that aims to eliminate some of the features of a voice disorder. This may result in further assessment as the diagnostic pic-ture becomes clearer.

ASSESSMENT OF VOCAL SYMPTOMS IN THE WORKPLACE

Problems relating to the use of voice at work are likely to arise in the classroom or lecture theatre, in the office, or in sports facilities. The basic principles of identifying whether there is a problem, investigating causes, and finding solutions are broadly similar and are based on risk assessment.

Hazard and Risk

Excess vocal load is hazardous – that is, it has the potential to cause harm. But it is the risk that harm will actually result that is important in the occupational health setting. Many people may undertake a hazardous activity, but few develop problems, perhaps because of individual resistance or because they do not do the hazardous activity for very long. Nevertheless, in the United Kingdom, health and safety law requires that employers identify hazards, evaluate risks, and put in control measures to reduce those risks as far as is reasonably practicable.

Several professions have been reported to be at high risk for voice disorders—these are outlined in Chapter 2. They include teaching, aerobics instruction, and acting. Anecdotal evidence from speech therapists suggests that they are seeing an increasing number of call center operators (Fig. 2) in their clinics; yet the literature on this group of workers is sparse. If there are a high number of call center workers treated to clinics (and there is no study suggesting this at present), then it could be due to one or more factors. As about 2% of the U.K. working population is now employed in call centers and the numbers are growing (Call Centre Association, personal communication, 2003), there is large population of workers, many of whom have voice problems as does the normal population. They may have jobs that are vocally demanding; any detriment causes difficulties at work, and so individuals present early. Conversely, there maybe a specific risk to the activity.

Indicators of Voice Disorder Risks

From an occupational perspective, there are several features that may indicate that there is a particular problem with a job or a working environment.

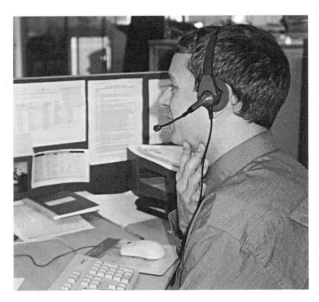

Figure 2   A Call center worker.

The way a job is designed in an office, sales environment, or call center may require the worker to use prolonged speech following a prepared script with few breaks. In a high-pressure environment requiring sales or contact targets to be met, there may be a lot of emotion and enthusiasm required to deliver information, which stresses the vocal apparatus. Workers may be required to work without breaks or access to drinks. There may be a need to shout to overcome background noise—for instance, in teaching or with poor environmental acoustics (e.g., aqua-aerobics instructors teaching a class from the side of a swimming pool). All these aspects of job and workplace design may contribute to the development of occupational voice disorders or may aggravate pre-existing voice problems.

Indicators of a Problem

There are several indicators that may suggest a problem with a task, job, or environment. These can be divided into reactive and proactive indicators.

Reactive Indicators

If staff are adequately trained to recognize that hoarseness or a weak voice can result from overuse and to report such symptoms early, then this reporting gives the best indication and opportunity to modify the aggravating factors and prevent further cases or progression of symptoms in an individual. An early reporting system is therefore fundamentally important.

Sickness absence records, early retirement cases, and civil claims are also indicators that need to be examined; however, compared to early reporting, they reflect problems that have been present for much longer.

Proactive Indicators

If a voice health problem is suspected, then a cross-sectional survey of workers' symptoms can be undertaken. A simple questionnaire has also been developed for use in such cases to allow the prevalence of voice symptoms to be assessed. A copy can be found in Appendix A. Completion times on average are only 4–5 minutes per person. While responses indicate the presence of voice dysfunction symptoms, as this is a cross-sectional instrument, they do not prove that any of the symptoms have been caused by any task, job, or environment. The results from groups of workers, however, can be used to compare working populations (e.g., voice symptoms in two offices of the same company) and changes in a single population over time (e.g., after improving working conditions).

When conducting any study of voice symptoms, it is important to remember that there will always be a background of people with voice disorder symptoms due to coughs, colds, use of medication, and pre-existing voice conditions. Studies looking at the prevalence of hoarseness, etc., are likely to find more cases in winter, when viral respiratory infections are more prevalent. Symptoms are also more likely to be present in populations with a high number of smokers or students/part-time workers who have part-time jobs in bars and clubs and so are exposed to smoke-filled atmospheres.

Determining Whether There Is Voice Health Problem in a Working Population

Establishing whether a group of workers are at risk of occupational voice disorders is achievable if several steps are taken.

First, management and worker representatives need to be engaged, a full explanation of the purpose of the study given, and how it will be carried out should be made clear.

An important area relates to the handling of data collected.

Key questions that need to be answered before any data are collected are:

1. What information will be collected?
2. Will it be anonymized?
3. What, if any, results will be passed to management?
4. What feedback will be given to the employer, worker representatives, and workers?
5. How will the data will be stored and destroyed?

6. How will participants be reassured that data collected will not be used for any other purpose?

In the United Kingdom, data need to be handled in compliance with both the Data Protection Act 1998 and guidance from the U.K. Information Commissioner (details are available from www.informationcommissioner.gov.uk). Ethical permission may also be needed if there is a proposed research element to the study.

Conducting a Study

Often, a presentation of the study to the group of workers is beneficial for recruitment to a study. This is not always possible because of the demands of the work, which is often paid on productivity: workers are thus reluctant to break away. Participation generally should be voluntary, and it is good practice that employers are not aware of those who decline to participate. Under the U.K. health and safety law, workers have a legal obligation to cooperate with employers if there is a health and safety issue, and so it is important to be clear at the outset whether this is a piece of research, information being gathered to contribute to a risk assessment, or an investigation into possible workplace health risks.

Analyzing Results

Once completed, questionnaires can be analyzed to identify whether specific groups of workers have problems. This can then lead to discussion with the group as to what they believe the problem is and what has caused it. It may be helpful to divide the possible causes into those related to:

- Workplace design (e.g., humidity, noise)
- Work design (e.g., long scripts)
- Worker behavior (e.g., poor posture, smoking)

Further investigation could lead to measurement of ambient humidity and noise levels or to redesign of a prepared script or rearrangement of pupils in a classroom.

ADVANCED WORKPLACE ASSESSMENT:
MEASUREMENT OF VOCAL LOADING

It has been estimated in Finland that approximately one-fourth of the total Finnish labor force work in professions that require the use of voice (46). Similar statistics have been presented for the United States (47). The largest groups of voice users consist of persons working in business and in teaching professions. Other large groups consist of telephone operators, military personnel, and clergy. Smaller groups important from the point of view of voice use are radio and TV staff as well as singers and actors (46). In addition, there are industrial workers whose tasks include voice use at high levels of background noise when giving instructions, for instance, which may place their vocal health at risk (see Refs. 48, 49 for reviews). There is substantial evidence implying that there is a causal relationship between vocal load at work and occupational voice disorders (see Refs. 48, 49 for reviews).

The total vocal workload consists of the individual and combined effects of various loading factors, shown in Table 1, which may also appear as occupational health hazards and risks. As gender and psychosocial and personality factors

Table 1 Vocal Loading Factors and Individual Cofactors Influencing Coping with Vocal Workload

Loading factors
Duration of voice use
Background noise level
Room acoustics
Quality of air
Other ergonomics
Psychosocial

Individual cofactors
Gender
Endurance
Health condition
Life habits
Vocal skill and experience
Psychosocial and personality

influence voice production at all levels, they are excluded from the figure.

Different methods have been developed for measuring loading at the level of vocal organ in field conditions. So far, the methods have been used for research purposes only. As to the different ways of collecting data of long-term voice use in field conditions, the methods can basically be divided into two groups: (1) audio recordings made in the field with digital recorders and analyzed with laboratory computers (50–63), and (2) portable microprocessors with analysis programs storing the results of the analyses, called dosimeters or voice accumulators. The following preset parameters have been measured: time and fundamental frequency (F0) (64); time and sound level (SL) (65–69); and time, F0, and SL (70,71). The major advantage of the aforementioned approach is that the laboratory analyses of the field recordings are not limited in any way, whereas the major drawback is that the analysis process can be very laborious and time-consuming. The opposite holds true for the portable microprocessor-based methods (63). At present, we do not know which parameters should be used to depict vocal function in the occupational context. Hence, using preset acoustic parameters may be problematic.

Using a microphone for recordings causes the problem of distinguishing between the subject and background noise and other speakers in the analysis. This can be solved to some extent by using short mouth-to-microphone distance (51), by doing manual corrections during the analysis phase (51), by using two microphones for phase difference detection (61), or by estimating the stationarity of the signal (60).

Accelerometers have been used as sensors as well (70,71). The advantage of the accelerometer over the microphone is that it is insensitive to background noise. On the other hand, its calibration for sound pressure level (SPL) analysis is not a simple task.

Specifically in the context of loading-related voice changes taking place during a working day, it seems that the only way of detection is through audio recordings to ensure that the samples chosen for comparison represent comparable speech situations. The analysis of the audio recordings can be made easier by reducing the length of the samples. In this case, however, the estimate of the total loading during the working day is very rough if the working task is not monotonous. One additional advantage of the use of audio recordings is that it permits traditional perceptual analyses of the samples. On the other hand, when a measure of the total vocal load during the day including pauses at work and leisure time is sought for, the use of dosimeters or accumulators seems necessary for legal and ethical reasons.

In addition to number of vocal fold vibrations (F0) and output level (SPL), the acoustical signal can be used to estimate the phonatory features and vibratory characteristics of the vocal folds by spectral analysis. Spectral parameters based on determination of the relationship between the energy level of lower and higher spectral components have been found to reflect voice changes caused by vocal loading (52,60).

The voice analysis results of loading examinations in the field can be further elaborated. One possibility is to combine the phonation time and F0 data, which gives the number of vocal fold vibrations. This has been called the vocal loading index (50). Svec et al. (70) have postulated relevant vocal doses: the time dose, the cycle dose, and the distance dose. The time dose is equal to the phonation (F0) time, and the cycle dose measures the total number of cycles accomplished by the vocal folds (vocal loading index) (50). The distance dose measures the total distance traveled by the vocal folds on their mediolateral oscillations. The distance dose is sensitive to both the frequency of oscillation of the vocal folds and the vocal output because the estimated amplitude of the vocal folds changes with the vocal output. Svec et al. (70) have estimated that the safety limits set for vibrating handheld tools (520 m accumulated distance per working day) are exceeded in less than one hour while speaking at a comfortable level.

In laboratory loading tests, it is possible to use, in addition to acoustic analyses, a wider variety of physiological methods, e.g., electromyographic recordings of the external frame musculature (46,72). Aerodynamic parameters, such as air flow (73) and subglottal pressure (74), have also been measured for research purposes. In clinical work, the value of laboratory vocal loading tests is questionable, especially because simulating heavy real-life vocal loading is difficult and can even be unethical.

As to other measurements of the loading factors set by the working task and present in the working environment, the principles of background noise measurements are well established (75,76). Reverberation time and speech transmission measurements are probably not often performed by occupational safety and health (OSH) personnel, but as they are important from the point of view of both the speaker and the listeners, their use as a routine part of any examination of the working conditions of voice and speech professionals should be considered. Rasti measurement is a subtype of the speech transmission index (77). It is a commercially available method that measures speech in two third-octave bands, centered at 500 Hz and 2 kHz. It uses a speechlike excitation signal and correlates modulation depth to loss of intelligibility. The deterioration of intelligibility is mainly a problem for the listener, but in an interactive situation, it will lead to repetitions and probably to louder voice use by the speaker to improve the penetration of the message.

Regarding air quality, measurement of humidity is a simple task, and a hygrometer should be included in the standard equipment in rooms predominantly used for speaking and singing. Analyses of dusts, molds, vapors, fumes, mists, etc., call for special methods (78,79) which, however, are usually available at OSH institutions.

The general principles of speech and singing training are the basis for observations concerning other ergonomic aspects (e.g., posture) of the work place of voice and speech professionals. In addition, the use, quality, and condition of voice amplifiers (80), if any, should be included in the observations. To the best of our knowledge, there are no checklists that can be used in on-site examinations of the working conditions of voice and speech professionals.

The principles of work-related psychosocial stress analyses and prevention are well developed within the OSH systems, and there are a plethora of methods and approaches from which to choose (81).

The methods of surveying the working conditions of voice and speech professionals are not well established, at least as far as voice analyses are concerned. The choice of appropriate method will depend on the purpose of the examination. For instance, for clinical purposes, audio recordings and perceptual analysis may be sufficient. However, in most cases, instrumental analysis is necessary. When an overall picture of the vocal load is sought, some kind of an accumulator no doubt is the instrument of choice, especially if in the future safety limits of tolerable occupational voice use can be developed. All in all, the development of the field of occupational voice disorders calls for cooperation between voice clinicians and OSH specialists.

REFERENCES

1. Carding PN. Voice pathology in the United Kingdom. BMJ 2003; 327:514–515.

2. Mathieson L. The Voice and Its Disorders. 6th ed. London: Whurr, 2001.

3. Harris T, Harris S, et al. The Voice Clinic Handbook. London: Whurr, 2000.

4. Dworkin JP, Meleca RJ. Vocal Pathologies: Diagnosis, Treatment and Case Studies. San Diego, CA: Singular, 1997.

5. Freeman M, Fawcus M. Voice Disorders and Their Management. London: Whurr, 2000.

6. Colton RH, Casper JK. Understanding Voice Problems: A Physiological Perspective for Diagnosis and Treatment. 2nd ed. Baltimore, MD: Williams and Wilkins, 1996.

7. Gleeson M, ed. Scott and Brown's Otolaryngology and Head and Neck Surgery. 10th ed. London: Arnold. In press.

8. Morrison M, Rammage L. The Management of Voice Disorders. London: Chapman and Hall Medical, 1994.

9. Carding PN. Measuring the Effectiveness of Voice Therapy. London: Whurr, 2000.

10. Jaconson BH, Johnson A, et al. The Voice Handicap Index (VHI): development and validation. Am J Speech Lang Pathol 1997; 6:66–70.

11. Deary I, Wilson JA, Carding PN, MacKenzie K. VoiSS: a patient derived Voice Symptom Scale. J Psychosom Res 2003; 54:483–489.

12. Rattenbury H, Carding PN. Evaluating the effectiveness and efficiency of voice therapy using trans-nasal laryngoscopy: a randomised controlled trial. J Voice. 2004; 18(4):522–533.

13. Verdolinni K, Hess MM, Titze IR, Bierhals W, Gross M. Investigation of vocal fold impact stress in human subjects. J Voice 1999; 13(2):184–202.

14. Baken RJ, Orlikoff RE. Clinical Measurement of Speech and Voice. 2nd ed. San Diego, CA: Singular, 2000.

15. Carding PN, Wade A. Managing dysphonia caused by misuse and overuse. BMJ 2000; 276:1544–1545.

16. McNeil MR, Rosenbeck JC, Aronson AE. The Dysarthrias: Physiology, Acoustics, Perception and Management. San Diego, CA: College-Hill Press, 1984.

17. Jurik AG, Pederson U, Norgard A. Rheumatoid arthritis of the cricoarytenoid joints: a case of laryngeal obstruction due to acute and chronic joint changes. Laryngoscope 1985; 95:846.

18. Teitel AD, MacKenzie CR, Stern R, Paget SA. Laryngeal involvement in systemic lupus erythematosus. Semin Arthritis Rheum 1992; 22:203–214.

19. Livesey J, Carding PN. Puberphonia or the male voice that will not break. Aust Voice 1996; 8:34–38.

20. Abitol J, de Brux J, Millot G, et al. Does a hormonal vocal cord cycle exist in women? Study of vocal pre-menstrual syndrome in voice performers by videostroboscopy–glottography and cytology on 38 women. J Voice 1989; 3:157–162.

21. Flach M, Schwickardi H, Simon R. What influence do menstruation and pregnancy have on a trained singing voice? Folia Phoniatr 1969; 21:199–200

22. Sataloff RT. Professional Voice: The Science and Art of Clinical Care. New York, NY: Raven Press, 1991.

23. Ritter FN. The effects of hyperthyroidism upon the ear, nose and throat. Laryngoscope 1967; 77:1427–1428.

24. Allen GW. Neoplasms of the thyroid gland. In: English GM, ed. Otolaryngology. New York, NY: Harper and Row, 1984.

25. Bone RC, Feren AP, Nahum AM. Laryngeal papillomatosis: immunologic and viral basis for therapy. Laryngoscope 1976; 86:341–346.

26. Goldberg J, Kovarsky J. Beclomethasone dipropionate inhalation treatment for chronic hoarseness in rheumatic disease. Arthritis Rheumatol 1983; 26:1412–1415.

27. Watkin K, Ewanowski S. Effects of aerosol corticosteroids on the voice: triamcinolone, acetonide and beclomethasone dipropionate. J Speech Hear Res 1985; 28:301–305.

28. Clarke PM, Durham SR, Perry A, MacKay IS. Objective measurement of voice change caused by inhaled steroids. Voice 1992; 1:63–66.

29. Koschkee DL, Rammage L. Voice Care in the Medical Setting. San Diego, CA: Singular, 1997.

30. Titze I. Biomechanics and distributed mass models of vocal fold vibration. In: Stevens KN, Hirano M, eds. Vocal Fold Physiology. Tokyo: University of Tokyo Press, 1981.

31. Gray SD, Hirano M, Sato K. Molecular and cellular structure of vocal fold tissue. In: Titze IR, ed. Vocal Fold Physiology: Frontiers of Basic Science. San Diego, CA: Singular, 1993.

32. Child DR, Johnson TS. Preventable and non-preventable causes of voice disorders. Semin Speech Lang 1991; 12:1–13.

33. Oates J. Chapter 7. In: Freeman M, Fawcus M, eds. Voice Disorders and Their Management. London: Whurr, 2000.

34. Lieberman J. Chapter 6. In: Harris T, Harris S, et al., eds. The Voice Clinic Handbook. London: Whurr, 2000.

35. Morrison M, Rammage L, Emami AJ. The irritable larynx syndrome. J Voice 1999; 13:447–455.

36. Koufman J. Reflux and voice disorders. In: Rubin J, et al., eds. Diagnosis and Treatment of Voice Disorders. New York, NY: Igaku-Shoin, 1995.

37. Forrest LA, Weed H. Candida laryngitis appearing as leukoplakia and GERD. J Voice 1998; 12:91–95.

38. Ramig LO, Verdolini K. Treatment efficacy: voice disorders. J Speech Lang Hear Res 1998; 41:S101–S166.

39. Wilson JA, Deary IJ, Millar A, MacKenzie K. The quality of life impact of dysphonia. Clin Otolaryngol. In press.

40. Ryan EB, Giles H, Sebastian RJ. An integrative perspective for the study of attitudes towards language variation. In: Ryan EB, Giles H, eds. The Social Psychology of Language. London: Edward Arnold, 1982.

41. Scherer K. Expression of emotion in voice and music. J Voice 1995; 9:235–248.

42. Moses PJ. The Voice of Neurosis. New York, NY: Grune and Stratton, 1954.

43. White A, Deary IJ, Wilson JA. Psychiatric disturbance and personality traits in dysphonic patients. Eur J Disord Commun 1997; 32:307–314.

44. Gudykunst WB. Intergroup communication. In: Giles H, ed. The Social Psychology of Language and Communication Studies. London: Edward Arnold, 1986.

45. Scherer K, Giles, H. Social Markers in Speech. Cambridge: Cambridge University Press, 1979.

46. Laukkanen A-M. On Speaking Voice Exercises. Ph.D. thesis, University of Tampere, Tampere, 1995.

47. Titze IR, Lemke J, Montequin D. Populations in the U.S. workforce who rely on voice as a primary tool of trade. NCVS Status Prog Rep 1996; 10:127–132.

48. Vilkman E. Occupational risk factors and voice disorders. Logop Phoniatr Vocol 1996; 21:137–141.

49. Vilkman E. Occupational safety and health aspects of voice and speech professionals. Folia Phoniatr Logop 2004.

50. Rantala L. Voice at Work [in Finnish]. Doctoral dissertation, University of Oulu, Oulu, 2000.

51. Rantala L, Haataja K, Vilkman E. Practical arrangements of a field examination of teachers' voice use. Scand J Log Phoniatr 1994; 19:43–54.

52. Rantala L, Paavola L, Körkkö P, Vilkman E. Working-day effects on the spectral characteristics of teaching voice. Folia Phoniatr Logop 1998; 50:205–211.

53. Rantala L, Vilkman E. Relationship between subjective voice complaints and acoustic parameters in teacher's voice. J Voice 1999; 13:484–495.

54. Rantala L, Vilkman E, Bloigu R. Voice changes during work: subjective complaints and objective measurements for female primary and secondary schoolteachers. J Voice 2002; 16: 344–355.

55. Jonsdottir V, Rantala L, Laukkanen A-M, Vilkman E. Effects of sound amplification on teachers' speech while teaching. Logop Phoniatr Vocol 2001; 26:118–123.

56. Jonsdottir V, Laukkanen A-M, Vilkman E. Changes in teachers' speech during a working day with and without electric sound amplification. Folia Phoniatr Logop 2002; 54:282–287.

57. Jonsdottir VI. The Voice: An Occupational Tool. Doctoral dissertation, University of Tampere, Tampere, 2003, http://acta.uta.fi.

58. Vilkman E, Lehto L, Bäckström T, Alku P. Vocal loading of call centre personnel. In: Schade G.

59. Schade G, Müller F, Wittenberg T, Hess M, eds. AQL 2003, Hamburg. Advances in Quantitative Laryugology, Voice and Speech Research. Proceedings Papers. Stuttgart: IRB Verlag, 2003. CD ROM, ISBN: 3–8167–6285–9. http://www.uke.uni-hamburg.de/AQL2003.

60. Bäckström T, Lehto L, Alku P, Vilkman E. Automatic presegmentation of running speech improves the robustness of several acoustic voice measures. Logop Phoniatr Vocol 2003; 28: 101–108.

61. Södersten M, Granqvist S, Hammarberg B, Szabo A. Vocal behavior and vocal loading factors for preschool teachers at work studied with binaural DAT recordings. J Voice 2002; 16:356–371.

62. Szabo Leroy A. The Voice at Work. Evaluation of Methods for Voice Documentation with Focus on Daycare Centers. Licentiate thesis, Department of Clinical Science, Division of Logopedics and Phoniatrics, Stockholm 2004.

63. Szabo A, Hammarberg B, Granqvist S, Södersten M. Methods to study the pre-school teacher's voice at work: simultaneous recordings with a voice accumulator and a DAT recorder. Logop Phoniatr Vocol 2003; 28:29–39.

64. Ohlsson A-C. Voice and Work Environment. Ph.D. thesis, University of Gothenberg, Gothenberg, 1988.

65. Masuda T, Ikeda Y, Manako H, Komiyama S. Analysis of vocal abuse: fluctuations in phonation time and intensity in 4 groups of speakers. Acta Otolaryngol (Stockh) 1993; 113:547–552.

66. Buekers R. Voice Performances in Relation to Demands and Capacity. Development of a Quantitative Phonometric Study of the Speaking Voice. Doctoral dissertation, University of Maastricht, Maastricht, 1998.

67. Buekers R, Bierens E, Kingma H, Marres EHMA. Vocal load as measured by the voice accumulator. Folia Phoniatr Logop 1995; 47:252–261.

68. Airo E, Olkinuora P, Sala E. A method to measure speaking time and speech sound pressure level. Folia Phoniatr Logop 2000; 52:275–288.

69. Sala E, Airo E, Olkinuora P, Simberg S, Ström U, Laine A, Pentti J, Suonpää J. Vocal loading among day care center teachers. Logop Phoniatr Vocol 2002; 27:21–28.

70. Svec JG, Titze IR, Popolo PS. Vocal dosimetry: theoretical and practical issues. In: Schade G, Müller F, Wittenberg T, Hess M, eds. AQL 2003, Hamburg. Advances in Quantitative Laryugology, Voice and Speech Research. Proceedings Papers. Stuttgart: IRB Verlag, 2003. CD ROM, ISBN: 3–8167–6285–9. http://www.uke.uni-hamburg.de/AQL2003.

71. Hillman R, Cheyne H. A portable vocal accumulator with biofeedback capability. In: AQL 2003, Hamburg. Advances in Quantitative Laryugology, Voice and Speech Research. Proceedings Papers. Stuttgart: IRB Verlag, 2003. CD ROM,

ISBN: 3–8167–6285–9. http://www.uke.uni-hamburg.de/ AQL2003.

72. Pettersen V, Westgaard RH. Muscle activity in the classical singer's shoulder and neck region. Logop Phoniatr Vocol 2002; 27:169–178.

73. Neils LR, Yairi E. Effects of speaking in noise on vocal fatigue and vocal recovery. Folia Phoniatr 1987; 39:104–112.

74. Vilkman E, Lauri E-R, Alku P, Sala E, Sihvo M. Effects of prolonged oral reading on F0, SPL, subglottal pressure, and amplitude characteristics of glottal flow waveforms. J Voice 1999; 13:303–315.

75. ISO. Ergonomic assessment of speech communication. Part I. ISO 9921-1, 1996.

76. Bruce RD, Bommer AS, Moritz CT. Noise, vibration, and ultrasound. In: DiNardi SR, ed. The Occupational Environment—Its Evaluation and Control. Fairfax: AIHA Press, 1997: 424–489.

77. Pekkarinen E, Viljanen V. Acoustic conditions for speech communication in classrooms. Scand Audiol 1991; 20:257–263.

78. Richter B, Löhle E, Knapp B, Weikert M, Schlömicher-Thier J, Verdolini K. Harmful substances on the opera stage: possible negative effects on singer's respiratory tracts. J Voice 2002; 16:72–80.

79. Cullen MR, Kreiss K. Indoor air quality and associated disorders. In: Levy BS, Wegman DH, eds. Occupational Health. 4th ed. Philadelphia: Lippincott Williams and Wilkins, 2000: 447–458.

80. McGlashan J, Howard D. Theoretical and practical considerations in the occupational use of voice amplification devices. In: Dejonckere P, ed. Occupational Voice—Care and Cure. The Hague: Kugler, 2001:165–186.

81. Baker DB, Karasek RA. Stress. In: Levy BS, Wegman DH, eds. Occupational Health. 4th ed. Philadelphia: Lippincott Williams and Wilkins, 2000:419–436.

5

Prevention and Treatment

PREVENTION AND TREATMENT IN THE CLINICAL SETTING

Prevention

Despite the growing evidence of an increasing incidence of voice problems among professional voice users, initiatives to prevent occurrence are very sporadic and poorly reported. For example, Martin (1) points out the paradox that teacher competency requires an ability to communicate clearly and effectively, and yet training rarely includes voice care strategies. This is even more nonsensical given our knowledge of vocal attrition in this professional group (2–4). Ramig and Verdolini (5) estimate that approximately 25% of the working population have jobs that critically require voice use. However, they also note that there is little proof of any formal or compulsory voice problem preventative initiatives for these workers. Furthermore, there is very little proof about the effectiveness of voice problem prevention programs in the research literature per se. Lehto et al. (6) reported the effects of a 2-day vocal training course on call center customer service advisors. They concluded that even a short vocal training program appeared to positively affect the self-reported vocal health of persons working in a vocally-demanding occupation. The authors acknowledge the need to expand the program to examine the effects on a larger number of nonselected workers over a longer time frame.

Information on how to manage the causes of voice problems (e.g., vocal misuse, vocal demand) is generally considered to be beneficial in helping professionals avoid a voice problem (7). We also know that voice therapy programs that aim to modify and manage the maintaining and prolonging features of a voice disorder have been shown to be effective (8–11). However, these studies commonly report on subjects who have already developed a voice disorder (and who are already attending for voice therapy). These principles could feasibly be incorporated into a preventative voice program along with other features seen as important to the relevant professional group (12). Longitudinal studies are required to assess how useful these programs are in preventing voice problems from occurring in these high-risk vocal groups.

Treatment

Clinical treatment of a voice problem falls into two main categories:

    a. Medical and surgical treatment
    b. Voice (speech) therapy and other conservative treatments

As described in Chapter 4, appropriate treatment depends on an accurate diagnosis and is best managed within a multidisciplinary environment (13). The two categories listed here should not be seen as mutually exclusive. It is possible for both treatment approaches to be conducted concurrently [e.g., medication for laryngo-pharyngeal reflux and voice therapy for hyperfunctional (strained) voice production]. It is also common for the two treatments to be planned consecutively. For example, a large majority of surgical procedures on the vocal apparatus will require postoperative voice therapy. Similarly, voice therapy may be indicated prior to surgery to eliminate compensatory vocal behaviors. In some cases, this may mean that surgery is avoided.

Surgical and Other Medical Treatments

Phonosurgery is the term used to describe laryngeal surgery, whose primary aim is the best possible restoration of laryngeal function and voice quality (13,14). Most laryngology surgeons would shy away from operating on a professional voice user's larynx unless it were absolutely necessary. This is probably a good thing because poorly executed phonosurgery may result in making the voice problem worse rather than better.

There are a number of benign laryngeal pathologies that are likely to require surgical intervention. These are detailed in Table 1.

Most of these surgical procedures require specialist phonosurgical techniques and instruments. Phonosurgery has become an established subspecialty within the general specialty of otolaryngology. The main principle underpinning all phonosurgical procedures appears to be the preservation (or restoration) of the superficial layers of the "lamina propria" (the layer between the surface epithelium and the vocal muscles). As described in Chapter 1, normal voicing requires a vertical waveform vibration of the mucosal edges of the vocal folds. Hence, phonosurgery attempts to deal with the underlying lesion while enabling these vibratory characteristics to occur once the healing process is complete (13).

There is some dispute about the appropriateness of surgical intervention for some benign pathologies of the vocal folds. Clearly, the skill of the surgeon is paramount in this decision. A careful examination and case history (by the whole voice clinic team) is imperative to ascertain the cause and maintaining factors of a vocal lesion. Surgical removal of a

Table 1 Benign Laryngeal Pathologies Commonly Requiring Surgical Intervention

Laryngeal pathology	Brief description
Vocal nodules	Mucosal thickening produced by damage to the basement membrane and situated at the junction of the anterior and mid-third of the vocal folds. Almost always bilateral.
Vocal polyps	Inflammatory epithelial lesions that are sessible or pedunculated and variable in size. Unilateral but sometimes with contralateral "contact" lesions.
Reinke's edema	A form of chronic laryngitis with typical bulky fold edge. Principally associated with smoking.
Epidermoid and retention cysts	A family of cysts that are mainly glandular in origin and that commonly contain mucus. Can vary in size, position, and specific histological characteristics.
Sulcus vocalis	A congenital variety of epidermoid cysts that have stretched along the length of the vocal fold and produced a furrow-like pocket along the fold.
Anterior laryngeal web	An adhesion of the laryngeal mucosa at the very anterior portion of folds.
Vergeture	An area of vocal ligament covered by a little scar tissue and atrophic epithelium. Suggested to be an acquired lesion (postsurgery?).

Source: From Ref. 13.

lesion will not resolve a problem which is essentially caused by vocal abuse, poor vocal hygiene, or other disease processes (i.e., laryngo-pharyngeal reflux). Bouchayer and Cornut (14) suggest a number of factors to be considered prior to surgery for vocal nodules (perhaps the commonly disputed lesion requiring surgical intervention). These are:

- The size and age of the lesion
- The failure of other medical and speech therapy treatments
- The impact of the lesion on stroboscopic examination (see Chapter 1)

- The objective and subjective importance of the problem to the patient

For a more detailed discussion of the indications and techniques of phonosurgery, the reader is directed to core texts such as References 13 and 14.

Pharmacological treatments for vocal problems clearly relate to the patient's presenting symptoms. There are many over-the-counter medications for "hoarse voice." However, evidence for the effectiveness is extremely poor. It is likely that most act as a mild anesthetic and nothing more. Harris et al. (13) summarize the types of common drugs used in laryngology practice as:

- Drugs that affect coughing and viscosity of mucous
- Drugs that modify allergic or asthmatic symptoms
- Anti-inflammatory drugs
- Bronchodilators
- Antibiotics
- Antacid medications

It should be noted that this list is of drugs used to help treat a voice problem (or a component). However, a number of these drugs may have adverse side affects. For example, antihistamines prescribed for reducing allergic symptoms can cause dryness with reduction and thickening of secretions (15). Drugs used for treating other conditions may deleteriously affect the voice (e.g., steroid inhalers for asthma). For a comprehensive review, the reader is directed to in-depth studies (13,15,16).

Voice Therapy Principles and Techniques

Voice therapy is a complex process that requires considerable skill from the clinician and significant motivation and insight from the patient. While voice therapy may follow a number of general principles, the specific treatment program will be customized to the individual patient's needs and expectations (8–10). It is the clinician's task to select appropriate techniques to match these needs and expectations and to enable the patient to achieve maximal vocal rehabilitation in the most efficient and effective manner. The evidence base for the effectiveness of voice therapy for most nonorganic voice disorders is reasonably strong (5,17,18). A number of studies using a variety of methodologies report positive outcomes (8–11). For simplification, voice therapy techniques are commonly classified into two categories: indirect and direct treatment approaches. In practice, these therapeutic techniques are frequently used simultaneously or at least in juxtaposition. Some of the most common ones are described briefly here. More details about technique rationale and administration are available from more comprehensive texts and published therapy programs (for review, see Ref. 15).

Indirect Treatment Approaches

The aim of these indirect techniques is to manage the contributory and maintenance aspects of a voice problem. Indirect approaches are based on the assumption that inappropriate phonatory behavior is a symptom of excessive vocal demands, vocally abusive behaviors, personal anxiety and tension, and a lack of knowledge of healthy voice production (17). The techniques include the following.

Education and Explanation: All patients need an appropriate working knowledge of normal phonatory behavior and how their own voice production differs from this. This places the rest of the treatment program in context and is likely to positively affect the patient's motivation and compliance. Patient understanding of the nature of their voice problem can also help reduce anxiety and establish positive and proactive attitude to vocal rehabilitation. It is also important for the professional voice user to feel "understood" by the clinician at a time of personal and professional vulnerability. The significant psychological, social, and economic impact of having a voice disorder should not be underestimated (1).

Vocal Tract Care/Vocal Hygiene: Appropriate levels of vocal care and attention to vocal hygiene are a vital step in vocal rehabilitation. This enables the patient to reflect on aspects of vocal abuse and misuse as well as observe healthy vocal habits such as adequate hydration and avoidance of laryngeal irritants. A number of vocal hygiene/care programs exist in the literature (for example, Ref. 15).

Voice Rest/Conservation: These approaches, which can clearly be as strict or general as necessary, are usually used in cases of vocal fold trauma or in the early days of postvocal fold surgery. Limiting vocal use obviously reduces the changes of mechanical damage of vocal fold vibration and allows spontaneous mucosal lining healing. Voice conservation is less strict than total voice rest and concentrates upon gentle/nonabusive modes of voice production that need to be clearly defined by the clinician and practiced by the patient.

Auditory Awareness: Many authors describe the need to "train" the voice patients' auditory skills to help them identify the undesirable features of their voice quality. This may be done by repeated analysis of high quality taped recordings. The rationale is that by monitoring the auditory output, the patient can begin to voluntarily control the unconscious function (15). The same principle is used to develop proprioceptive awareness of voice production.

Relaxation: General relaxation techniques may be used to enable patients to be able to focus on their own body and mechanisms of voice production without the distractions of daily life. Specific techniques can target muscle groups to reduce their tension and hence improve the movement, coordination, and flexibility of the muscle of phonation. Reducing articulator and jaw tension may require specific exercises. These methods may be particularly useful for voice users in stressful jobs or those placed in vocally stressful situations (e.g., telephone sales, motivational speakers).

Posture: Poor body posture is likely to restrict breathing and contribute to muscle tension (13). Particular attention should be paid to habitual postural demands in the workplace where regular voice use is also required (1). Some of these aspects are discussed later in this chapter.

Breath Support: Deep and regular diaphragmatic breathing is a prerequisite for good voice production.   Particular attention should be paid to the controlled expiratory flow of the air for voicing. Anxiety levels, physical activity (i.e., aerobic activity), and postural restrictions (including tight clothing) may all affect appropriate diaphragmatic breathing patterns.

Manual Therapy: Excessive tension in the intrinsic and extrinsic laryngeal muscles may also be reduced by manual massage and digital mobilization. A number of authors reported rapid success with these techniques in reducing laryngeal discomfort and laryngeal muscle tension (15,19).

Psychological Counseling: The patient's emotional and psychological status may be central to either the etiology or maintenance of the voice disorder. Many of these aspects can be addressed by the sensitive approach of a skilled clinician (15). Sometimes more specialist psychological help is required depending on the nature of the problem.

Direct Treatment Approaches

The aim of these approaches is to modify aspects of faulty voice to promote appropriate and efficient voice production. This attempt at treatment is based on the assumption that the patient has adopted incorrect and potentially damaging methods of phonation. The approaches include the following.

Reducing Vocal Strain: Excessive laryngeal effort during phonation is a common feature of the disordered voice. A wide range of exercises exist to counteract hyperfunctional phonation and help the patient achieve good vocal fold adduction with appropriate laryngeal effort (9–11,13,15).

Changing Voice Quality: With guidance from the clinician, the patient may change aspects of the method of voice production that, in turn, will alter the quality of the voice produced. In effect, the patient learns to modify breath support, air flow, vocal fold adduction/tension, and resonance to produce the desired acoustic effect. The subject must then learn to reproduce and habitualize these features by using auditory and kinesthetic feedback.

Pitch Modification: A disordered voice may present with a habitual pitch that is either too high or too low. Experimentation with different vocal pitches frequently results in desirable changes of laryngeal effort, perceived voice quality, and enhanced vocal resonance (15,20).

Breath Flow (Transglottic Air Flow): Improved control of the airflow that passes through the larynx and vibrates the vocal folds is likely to improve the regularity and stability of the resulting sound. Many clinic therapy programs emphasize the need for a controlled "power source," which in turn allows the vocal folds to vibrate without requiring constant modification because of variable transglottic air flow.

Breathing and Phonation Coordination: Coordination of breathing patterns with voicing is important for connected speech. Awareness and skilled execution of how to use two features in combination can be developed by using exercises concerned with phrase length, intentional pitch and volume changes, extended speaking demands, and so forth. This may help the patient generalize good vocal technique into more complex speaking tasks.

Enhanced Resonance: Improving vocal resonance enables the speaker to maximize voice quality and carrying power. Furthermore, the sensory and auditory feedback achieved in many resonance exercises enables the speaker to increase vocal loudness with minimum effort and with no additional hyperfunction. These skills can obviously be of great value for occupational voice users who require a loud voice (e.g., teachers, aerobic instructors, machine operators, and clergy).

Projection and Amplification: Many professional voice users require additional work on aspects of voice projection and voice amplification. Appropriate voice projection requires a good breathing-for-speech technique, a relaxed (minimal effort) laryngeal vibratory mechanism, and an open oral tract that is able to maximally resonant the sound. In addition, clear and precise articulation is essential for audibility in large and/ or noisy spaces. A number of voice amplification systems are now available, and these can range from small lectern microphones to portable (i.e., attached to a belt) amplifiers with tie-pin microphones to hands-free microphones (often seen with aerobic instructors).

These speech-and-voice therapy treatment techniques cannot be done in an isolated clinical setting without also addressing the specific work environment and context for the voice user.

PREVENTION, TREATMENT, AND MANAGEMENT IN THE WORKPLACE

General Principles of Prevention

The prevention of occupational voice disorders requires a pro-active systematic approach involving management, employees, and professional health and safety advisors.

Key to prevention is risk assessment. Risk assessment is a process whereby a competent person identifies the hazards involved in a particular task or activity, evaluates the risk of developing ill health or having an accident from carrying out that activity, and puts into place control measures to reduce the risk of such accidents or ill health. But this is not the end of the process. Risk assessments should be regularly reviewed to ensure that the assumptions made about the level of risk and the controls needed remain adequate. Review should also take place after a change in a particular task (e.g., the introduction of a new script for telesales workers in a call center or a move to larger classrooms for a teacher).

An introduction to the principles of risk assessment can be found in a leaflet which can be downloaded from the free leaflet section of the Health and Safety Executive (HSE) website at www.hse.gov.uk.

A basic checklist for assessing risks, vocal risks, and demands is provided in Appendix A. It is not meant to replace competent advice but aims to provide an idea of the type of assessment needed.

Risk Assessment

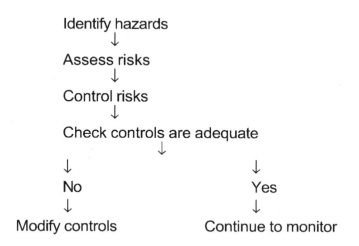

Identify hazards
↓
Assess risks
↓
Control risks
↓
Check controls are adequate
↓

↓	↓
No	Yes
↓	↓
Modify controls	Continue to monitor

Legal Framework

In the United Kingdom, employers have legal duties under the Health and Safety at Work Act 1974 (21) to do all that is reasonably practicable to ensure the health, safety, and welfare of their staff. Under the Management of Health and Safety at Work Regulations 1999, employees are required to carry out risk assessments and hence must identify hazards that arise from work, assess risks, and put in controls to ensure that ill health does not result from those work activities (22). Legislation also requires that employees be provided with information, instruction, and training on how to do their jobs safely (22) and that they cooperate with their employers in arrangements that are made for health and safety reasons (21). Specific regulations apply to the use of display screen equipment (23); these require an ergonomic risk assessment of workstations to be performed. This assessment must look at posture and eye and eyesight. Risk assessments should be holistic and cover all risks from a particular task or job and not just center on the risks to the voice.

Teachers, for example, not only suffer voice problems but may also experience violence from pupils and occupational stress. Risk factors for these conditions also need to be included in a comprehensive risk assessment.

Practical Steps in Prevention

To prevent occupational voice disorders, it is necessary to look at three areas: work design, workplace design, and the worker.

Work Design

The cornerstone of prevention is good work design. Often attention is only paid to how a job will be done, not how to make a job and environment easier to do that job in. Ideally, consideration of the needs of the voice user should be incorporated into the design stage of any work activity and workplace. Properly designed workspaces improve productivity and performance, and this in turn promotes improvements in workers' health.

For all voice users, consideration should be given to the following factors relevant to voice usage:

- the time spent speaking continuously;
- the need to incorporate breaks from talking and
- the volume of speech required to do the job while compensating for background noise, etc.

The task should be designed to:

1. Reduce the need to shout or use the voice continuously, e.g., by supplying teachers/lecturers with microphones and by collocating teams of workers together in a call center so that they do not shout to each other.
2. Avoid the risks for dysphonia, e.g., by providing readily accessible water to ensure hydration, and to train staff on vocal hygiene and how to avoid voice strain.
3. Reduce the length of time spent talking, e.g., by designing scripts where the client talks and there are adequate breaks, and ensuring that shift lengths do not lead to voice overuse.

Workplace Design

The general structure and layout of the workplace is the first important step in the prevention of voice problems. The design should take into account the voice usage and also reduce outside noise by using materials that absorb internal noise and by considering the vocal demands that are needed. Within the teaching environment, the arrangement of desks and chairs is likely to influence the degree to which voice projection is needed. The location of disruptive pupils may have to be managed to reduce shouting and projection, and alterations may need to be made to lecturers' teaching styles if they need to use a microphone because of weak voice.

Temperature

Correct temperature is important for worker comfort and for maximum productivity. In the United Kingdom, a reasonable working temperature would be around 19°C (24). Temperatures can be raised at workstations and desks near windows and by heat generated from electrical equipment such as printers and photocopiers. A high level of occupancy in a building, particularly working 24/7, also raises ambient temperatures, as does the pattern of use of the working space.

When temperature is thought to be a problem in a workplace, then it is important to have a measurement strategy, as within one room temperature can vary depending on the effects of radiant heat from the sun near windows, to localized heat from equipment and to changes in regulation because of unoccupied work areas, e.g., on night shifts some centers close down parts of buildings that then become cold and can alter the balance of the system.

Measuring Temperature: Temperature should be measured by ordinary dry bulb thermometer, close to the workstations and the workers. Measurements should be taken at working height and away from windows and local sources of heat.

What to do if There Are Problems with Temperature

- Fans and heaters can alleviate small spots of inequality and discomfort through too much or too little heat.
- Ideally install a system where workers optimize the temperature themselves rather than a centrally controlled system.
- Be aware of the effects of subsequently installing screens and barriers to airflow as these may affect temperature.
- Be aware that seasonal variations in temperature should be considered to maintain optimum comfort for workers.

Humidity

As discussed in an earlier chapter, the humidity of inspired air is very important for vocal health as dryness of the throat and vocal passages increases the risk of voice dysfunction.

Normal levels of humidity range from 40% to 70% (relative humidity) with the lower end more comfortable in warmer offices (24). These are general levels across a workplace, but it is important to be aware that pockets of low humidity can be caused by heat from computers and printers.

Often the first group of employees to notice either local or general low humidity are contact lens wearers who start to complain of dry and irritated eyes. Employees may also complain of dry mouths or sore throats. Low humidity dermatoses (rashes) have also been reported in the literature.

Measuring Humidity: A whirling hygrometer (similar in appearance to a football rattle) can be used to provide a snapshot of humidity levels; alternatively, continuous monitoring can be undertaken.

What to do if There Are Problems with Humidity

1. Rebalance the air conditioning system centrally.
2. Consider seasonal variations in humidity when planning checks on air conditioning.

Air Quality and Ventilation

For mechanical ventilation systems, the UK recommended minimum fresh airflow is $8\,L\ sec^{-1}$/person in no smoking areas, and air velocities should be around 0.1–0.15 m sec^{-1} in winter and up to 0.25 m sec^{-1} in summer (24). Levels greater than this may be perceived to be drafts. In the United Kingdom, Regulation 6 of the Workplace (Health, Safety, and Welfare) Regulations 1992 (25) requires employers to ensure that all workplaces should be ventilated either with fresh air from outside the building or with air that has been adequately filtered and purified. If there is a high level of occupancy (or 24-hour usage), then irritants can build up and the circulation rate needs to be increased.

Lighting

The level of lighting to do a particular task is very important to maintain good posture and prevent slouching. Poor lighting can make a worker difficult, increase the number of errors made, and reduce productivity. The following standards of lighthing for offices have been publised by architects and building designers (26).

- Minimum daylight factor > 0.5% and
- Average daylight factor > 2–5% (where daylight factor is the ratio of lux inside/lux outside × 100% and lux is a measurement of light).

Noise

Noise in the workplace, either generated by equipment, fellow workers, or pupils, can cause workers to shout over background noise to be heard. A study of background noise in call centers found the levels to be around 60 dB (J. Patel Health and Safety Laboratories, Sheffield, U.K., personal communication). Background and ambient noise can be reduced by good workplace design of collocating teams that need to exchange information, avoiding high ceilings, and using plants, foliage, and furnishings to dampen noise (although the efficacy of the latter has not been proven).

Dust and Cleanliness

Dust and dirt can act as a respiratory irritant; hence, it is important that workplaces in which there are high vocal demands remain clean and dust levels are reduced as far as possible. Because damp cleaning has been shown to reduce airborne dust levels, dry sweeping and dusting should be discouraged. In 24-hour workplaces, care must be taken when cleaning is carried out while work is in progress. Closing down sections, cleaning, and then reopening them may be a better approach.

U.K. government recommendations include that there be a clear reporting system for adverse environmental problems in workplaces such as call centers (27).

Workers

Finally, the worker is the most important aspect of occupational vocal health. Workers need to know that use of their voice at work, if not done correctly, can lead to short- and long-term problems. In the United Kingdom employers must provide information, instruction and training on work hazards and risks. Appendix B includes a list of topics which could be addressed in vocal health training programs. Such programs should include a brief description of how the voice works, the importance of hydration and the avoidance of irritants such as tobacco smoke, and the interaction and impact of common medications, including those that can be purchased without prescription. The importance of resting the voice, taking breaks, and reporting any early symptoms also need to be included.

Management of Voice Problems in the Workplace

Policy

Managing any occupational health risk depends on a well-organized and structured management system. Key to this is acknowledging the potential risks and clearly defining the roles and responsibilities of stakeholders. Critical players are likely to be the Board or Chief Executive who lends influence to the issue and allocates resources for proper management;

the line manager or supervisor who is responsible for carrying out risk assessments and actioning preventative advice and managing cases in a supportive atmosphere; the professional advisors (including occupational health physician or nurse) who advise the company and the employee on what needs to be done; and the workers themselves who have to be responsible for following company policies, reporting symptoms early, and following advice.

Other important players include the employee representatives and unions who can support the company policy and reinforce good practice, and the designers of work equipment and work systems who can design healthy work in a healthy environment.

A sample policy outlining a possible organization of responsibilities is shown in Appendix B. Each policy needs to be tailored to individual circumstances and company culture—one size does not fit all and the policy shown here is not intended to replace professional advice.

Risk Assessment

Having recognized the issue and drafted a policy, the company then needs to organize assessment of the risks involved. A brief checklist for identifying risks to voice health is shown in Appendix A. Risk assessment needs to be holistic and should include the effect of sustained or abnormal posture, stress-inducing work conditions or monitoring, poor work organization, unrealistic targets, and the degree of support and control workers have. Some guidance on identifying causes of stress in the workplace that can be incorporated in risk assessments can be found in the U.K. Health and Safety Executives, guidance on management standards for workplace stress (www.hse.gov.uk). Basic health and safety risks such as slips, trips, falls, violence, abusive behavior, and back pain also need to be considered depending on the work and workplace.

Risk Control

Having identified the risks, it is important to set mechanisms in place to control the risks. Depending on the work undertaken, this may mean reducing the length of pre-prepared scripts for telesales workers, decreasing targets, increasing the frequency (but not necessarily the overall length) of breaks for completed calls for call handlers, or arranging disruptive pupils at the front of a class to reduce the need to shout.

It is more successful to design preventative solutions than add them to existing ways of working. Hence, liaising with employees and developing a smoke-free workplace (with support for those smokers who wish to give up), installing water fountains where they are easily accessed, and ensuring close control of humidity are all important in preventing voice ill health and are relevant to all work settings.

Monitoring

Proactive risk management involves checking systems that are put in place to protect health and identifying whether things are going wrong, as quickly as possible, so that they can be remedied.

Monitoring for voice health problems (Appendix C) needs to be holistically undertaken with other health monitoring systems, and not in isolation.

Businesses and organizations should check whether their control of risks, which may impair voice health are adequate in protecting workers by:

- Checking sick notes (both from doctors and those completed by the employees themselves for shorter-term absences) for a voice-related problem;
- Asking employees to declare any problems at the start of a shift as a routine start to the work (this is habitually undertaken by some large automotive manufacturers twice a day);
- Providing posters and information around the workplace that encourage reporting of symptoms to line managers or occupational health staff.

If there is a suggestion of problems, then a simple questionnaire such as that shown in Appendix D can be used. Care should be taken, however, in interpretation as a cross-sectional assessment of symptoms does not mean that symptoms are caused by work. It just gives an idea of the extent of the problem and how many resources are needed to manage it.

Early Reporting and Training

Encouraging employees to report symptoms early is important in preventing more significant problems. The need to report should be included in introductory training and reinforced by supervisors and through other training opportunities, posters, and information around the workplace.

Rehabilitation and the Disability Discrimination Act 1995 (DDA)

If an individual has a vocally-demanding job but has a voice problem, then alternative duties need to be considered. It is important to try to keep the employee at work and engaged in work activities. Being away from work because of a voice problem can be necessary, but does occur at a cost of loss of contact with colleagues and lack of updating skills relevant to the job. Returning after a long absence, whatever the reason, can require rehabilitation with reduced hours, alternative duties, and change of tasks.

The DDA 1995 applied, until recently, to businesses employing more than 15 people. As of October 2004, the provisions have been extended to smaller workplaces and also specific groups such as police officers who were previously exempt. In simple terms, the DDA defines disability as a physical or mental impairment which affects an individual's ability to undertake activities of daily living. As such, it is likely to apply to people with voice disorders if the problem lasts 12 months or more. Whether a person is disabled under the meaning of the Act is determined not by occupational health physicians, but by the Employment Tribunals (ETs). If an employee is considered disabled, an employer must make reasonable adjustments to allow the person to work. Again, it is the ETs who decide what is reasonable and what is not. Cases heard so far suggest that adjustments to working hours, alternative less vocally demanding duties, or more frequent breaks may be considered reasonable for legal compliance.

REFERENCES

1. Martin S. Chapter 13. In: Freeman M, Fawcus M, eds. Voice Disorders and Their Management. Whurr, 2000.

2. Sapir S, Keidar A, Mathers-Schmidt B. Vocal attrition in teachers: survey findings. Eur J Disord Commun 1993; 28: 177–185.

3. Miller MK, Verdolini K. Frequency and risk factors for voice problems in teachers of singing and control subjects. J Voice 1995; 9(4):348–362.

4. Koufman JA, Blalock PD. Vocal fatigue and dysphonia in professional voice users; Bogart-Bacall syndrome. Laryngoscope 1988; 98:493–498.

5. Ramig LO, Verdolini K. Treatment efficacy: voice disorders. J Speech Hear Res 1998; 41:S101–S116.

6. Lehto L, Rantala L, Vilkman E, Alku P, Backstrom T. Experiences of a short vocal training course for call-center customer service advisors. Folia Phoniatrica Logopedics 2003; 55(4):163–176.

7. Mattiske JA, Oates JM, Greenwood KM. Vocal problems among teachers: a review of prevalence, cause, prevention, and treatment. J Voice 1998; 13(4):489–499.

8. Carding PN, Horsley IA, Docherty GJ. A study of the effectiveness of voice therapy in the treatment of 45 patients with non-organic dysphonia. J Voice 1999; 13:72–104.

9. Stemple JC, Lee L, Damico B, Pickup B. Efficacy of vocal function exercises as a method of improving voice production. J Voice 1994; 8:270–278.

10. MacKenzie K, Millar A, Sellars C, Wilson JA, Deary IJ. Is voice therapy an effective treatment for dysphonia? A randomised controlled trial. Br Med J 2001; 323:658–661.

11. Holmberg EB, Hillman RE, Hammarberg B, Sodersten M, Doyle P. Efficacy of a behaviorally based voice therapy protocol for vocal nodules. J Voice 2001; 15:395–412.

12. Yiu EM-L. Impact and prevention of voice problems in the teaching profession: embracing the consumer's view. J Voice 2002; 16(2):215–228.

13. Harris T, Harris S, et al. The Voice Clinic Handbook. London: Whurr, 2000.

14. Bouchayer M, Cornut G. Chapter 17. In: Freeman M, Fawcus M, eds. Voice Disorders and Their Management. Whurr, 2000.

15. Mathieson L. The Voice and its Disorders. 6th ed. London: Whurr, 2001.

16. Sataloff RT. Professional Voice: The Science and Art of Clinical Care. New York: Raven Press, 1991.

17. Carding PN. Measuring the Effectiveness of Voice Therapy. London: Whurr, 2000.

18. Carding PN, Hillman RE. More randomised controlled studies in speech and language therapy. Br Med J 2001; 323:645–646.

19. Roy N, Leeper HA. Effects of the manual laryngeal musculoskeletal tension reduction technique for functional voice disorders. J Voice 1993; 7:242–249.

20. Laguaite JK, Waldrop WF. Acoustic analysis of fundamental frequency of voice before and after therapy. N Z Speech Ther J 1963; 18:23.

21. Health and Safety at Work Act 1974. Statutory Instrument. London: HMSO, 1974.

22. Management of Health and Safety at Work Regulations 1999. Statutory Instrument. London: HMSO, 1999.

23. Health and Safety (Display Screen Equipment) Regulations 1992. Statutory Instrument. London: HMSO, 1992.

24. Health and Safety Executive How to Deal with Sick Building Syndrome. Guidance for Employers, Building Owners, and Building Managers. HSG 132, ISBN 0-71-76-0861-1.

25. Workplace (Health, Safety, and Welfare) Regulations 1992. Statutory Instrument No 3004. London: HMSO, 1992.

26. www.bco-officefocus.com/comfort. Accessed 8/11/2004.

27. Advice Regarding Call Center Practices. HSE/LA Enforcement Liaison Committee HELA, December 2001. www.hse.gov.uk/lau/lacs 94–1. Rev. accessed 17/12/2004.

6

Occupational Voice Disorders from a Legal Perspective: Civil Claims for Damages

Claims for damages for occupationally-induced illness/disease have been brought before the courts since the end of the 19th century. Legal actions for asbestos-related disease, occupationally-induced deafness, vibration white finger, repetitive strain injury, and, most recently, stress at work, to name but a few, are commonplace in the field of personal injury law. A brief review of volumes 3 and 4 of Kemp and Kemp's *The Quantum of Damages* (Sweet and Maxwell) reveals how frequently such claims are litigated.

There is now another category to be added to this formidable list, namely, claims arising out of occupationally-induced voice damage. In recent times, there has been recognition that employees like teachers and call center workers who are required to talk almost continuously throughout their working day are at a risk of suffering voice damage. While the mechanism by which the voice comes to be damaged is, of course, unique to its own physiological makeup, as a general proposition like any other part of the anatomy (such as an upper limb) excessive or overuse has the potential to cause damage.

Doubtless, voice clinicians have long been aware of the hazards associated with overuse or abuse of the voice. But it is only quite recently that information has been promulgated about the risks of damage consequent to excessive use of the voice. For example, it was not until 1994 that the Health and Safety Executive provided some guidance on safe working practices in call centers through the "Initial Advice Regarding Call Centre Working Practices" (LAC Number 94/1). This publication was revised in December 2001 (LAC Number 94/rev). It is reasonable to suppose that the problem has become somewhat more acute because of increased use of vocal communication in our working lives (e.g., presentations, telephones, video communication links). A good example is telephone banking. In 1997, the Banking, Finance and Insurance Union, in response to a number of complaints of voice loss among workers engaged in telephone banking, published an article entitled "Occupational Voice Loss: A Negotiator's Guide" (BIFU Research Department). Fortunately, because of such publications and some coverage in the media, there does now seem to be an increasing awareness of the need to take measures to guard against voice damage, especially in professions where employees talk continously during their working day.

While it is to be anticipated that within the next few years there will be a number of claims for damages for voice injuries (principally on the part of professional voice users), certain legal criteria need to be satisfied for such claims to succeed. The mere fact that an employee has suffered voice damage does not by itself give rise to entitlement to an award of damages. An employee seeking damages in such circumstances has to prove fault (negligence) on the part of

the employer and that damage has been sustained as a direct consequence of the employer's negligence (causation).

The concept of negligence is not straightforward, but contains a number of elements. First, it must be demonstrated that a work-related injury was reasonably foreseeable. Hence, if a factory worker were to suffer damage to his voice, even if in some way related to his work, it is unlikely that he would be able to pursue a claim for damages. This is because his employers could convincingly argue that a factory environment would not necessarily contribute to voice damage. The position is plainly otherwise when, for example, a teacher suffers voice damage. It is now well understood and presumed to be within the knowledge of employers, such as local authorities, that persons who use their voice throughout the day and who frequently raise their voice are at risk of suffering long-term damage. Accordingly, given the state of knowledge that now exists, the test of "reasonable foreseeability" is likely to be satisfied in cases where employees use their voice for long periods of time in the course of their work. The situation is, of course, far less clear with respect to environmental (atmospheric) conditions in the work place and how this may impact upon vocal health. The scientific evidence surrounding these controversies needs to be established before any legal proceedings can be contemplated.

The next stage is to demonstrate that there were steps that could have been reasonably taken by employers to protect their employees' voices. An obvious first step would be a program of education and information. Such a method ought to include warnings that voice damage can occur if appropriate precautions are not taken. Employees should be instructed as to what preventative measures can be taken properly (e.g., keep the throat lubricated, drink water rather than tea or coffee to maintain hydration, rest the voice whenever possible, and, especially, report any voice health problems to the occupational health team or medical practitioner). Call center workers, especially, should be told to break opening greeting scripts into shorter segments to give them frequent microbreaks, while callers respond to their questions. In the context of large employers where many employees are exposed to the risk of voice damage, it might be reasonable to expect that each of these employees is provided with some written information and guidance as how to best protect his/her voice.

Additionally, it may be reasonable to argue that employers (wherever reasonably practicable) should try to operate a system of job rotation, i.e., to intersperse tasks that involve continuous talking with other duties. This might be difficult in the teaching environment, but presumably it could be managed within a call center. Other measures would no doubt include ensuring that reasonable temperatures are maintained in the workplace with suitable ventilation.

If employers under some circumstances do not undertake such preventative measures where voice damage is foreseeable, then arguably negligence will be established. There may also be scope to debate whether the employers were in breach of various statutory regulations: for example, Regulation 6 of the Workplace (Health, Safety and Welfare) Regulations 1992 requires an employer make effective and suitable provision to ensure that work space is adequately ventilated by a sufficient quantity of fresh or purified air, while Regulation 7 imposes an obligation to ensure that temperatures in the workplace are reasonable.

However, with an increasing emphasis on matters of health and safety at work and a growing awareness of the potential for voice damage, it is to be expected that at least larger employers will put preventive measures in place. If they do so, and if an employee nevertheless suffers voice damage, then it will not be possible to prove negligence or breach of statutory duty, with the result that any claim on the part of an employee will fail. Moreover, it is worth emphasizing that an employer only needs to take reasonable steps to protect his employees from suffering injury. By way of illustration, an employer would not be expected to impose a regime of "water breaks": it would be deemed sufficient to advise employees to drink water regularly and to ensure that chilled drinking water is made available.

The nature and extent of the employers' duty would, however, change if they were put on notice that an employee was suffering some voice difficulties. In that event, an employer would need to be proactive, taking all necessary steps to minimize any risk of long-term damage. This might well necessitate transferring an employee to a different department or allocating tasks that do not involve prolonged use of the voice.

Once a claimant is in a position to establish negligence, it is then necessary to show that damage has ensued because of such a condition. This is both a medical and a legal issue. Medically, it will need to be shown that as a consequence of excessive use of the voice, damage has occurred. Thus, the claimant will need to be examined by a voice pathologist with a view to establishing a diagnosis of work-induced dysphonia (or vocal abuse in the work place). If in fact the complaint of voice damage is found to be because of infection, such as laryngitis, then plainly medical causation will not be established. On the other hand, if the voice specialist is able to say that, on the basis of probabilities, the dysphonia has been caused by excessive use of the voice, then the hurdle of causation is overcome. The clinical world is, however, rarely simple and, as is well known, many voice disorders begin as one problem (e.g., laryngitis) and develop into another (e.g., voice abuse). Again, it is incumbent upon the voice clinician to establish the relative contribution of the etiological factors.

In addition, legal causation needs to be proved. In the context of dysphonia, this is probably not a major obstacle for claimants. Specifically, it should be possible to demonstrate (with some input from the medical expert) that if an employer had complied with his duty to take reasonable steps to protect his employee's voice, then the injury would have been avoided or at least would have been much less serious. To put it in another way, it is sufficient, for example, to show that a failure to provide breaks for a call center worker for the purposes of resting her voice has made a material contribution to her dysphonia.

Nevertheless, an employer will have defense if it can be demonstrated that despite putting in place all reasonable measures and precautions, the claimant would have still suffered the same level of voice damage. Presumably such a situation could arise if there was a specific vulnerability or susceptibility to voice problems (e.g., if the claimant had a long and protracted history of voice problems prior to the present job or continued to engage in vocally abusive behavior outside of the workplace).

It is also necessary to reflect on the nature and extent of the damage. There is obviously a very wide spectrum: at one end of the scale, an employee may suffer a transient disturbance in her voice with no long-term term consequences, while at the other extreme there may be permanent and significant damage to the laryngeal structures. If the damage is temporary and is of a comparatively minor nature, then it would be difficult to justify a claim for damages. In such circumstances, damages would be measured in hundreds of pounds/dollars with the result that costs would far exceed the value of the claim. But at the other end of the scale, there could be a very substantial claim for pain, suffering, and disability, particularly if a person's voice has been permanently altered. For elite professional voice users for whom the quality of the vocal sound is extremely important (e.g., an opera singer), this can be a very serious matter indeed. There could also be an award to reflect loss of earnings and/or loss of ability to pursue a chosen career. With regard to the latter, it is not difficult to envisage circumstances where an employee may be advised to give up a particular employment because of a chronic voice condition. For some professional voice users (e.g., teachers, lawyers, clergymen, sales executives), this could result in an enforced career change, with all of the financial and personal consequences of retraining. However, claims where damages reach tens of thousands of pounds are likely to be comparatively rare.

For the record, the author, in the course of his work as a barrister specializing in personal injuries, has only been involved in one claim where damages were sought for occupationally-induced voice injury. The claim was on behalf of a female employee who worked at a customer service center. Over a three year period between 1997 and 2000, she spent the entire working week (37.5 hr) answering telephone calls from customers. The calls followed each other immediately with no gap in between. The only breaks were one hour for lunch and two 15 min breaks in the morning and afternoon, respectively. The employee developed an ache on the left side of the larynx, a feeling of choking/tightness, hoarseness, and from time to time a complete absence of voice. Eventually, she received treatment from a specialist speech therapist which had the desired effect.

A claim was initiated on the basis that the claimant had received no warnings about the risk of voice damage, nor had any preventative measures been put in place. Somewhat predictably, liability was denied on the basis that it was not foreseeable that the claimant would suffer injury to her voice because of answering the telephone, and, in any event, it was not accepted that any voice damage was work-related. Medical evidence was obtained and the expert was able to confirm a diagnosis of functional dysphonia because of excessive use of her voice during working hours. Eventually, after commencing proceedings, the defendant employer put forward an offer which was acceptable to the claimant. Damages were comparatively modest since the claimant had made a fairly good recovery, albeit she was advised not to undertake work which involved long periods talking on the telephone.

In conclusion, while it seems likely that this will be a growth area in the field of personal injury litigation, it is to be hoped that with increasing publicity, employers will take active steps to protect their employees' voices. If they do so, then it is likely that in the longer term, there will be fewer claims.

7

Resources

USEFUL WEBSITES

Voice Disorder/Voice Clinic Centers

a. New York Eye and Ear Infirmary Center for voice. http://www.nyee.edu/cfv.html.

    The website includes special section on professionals at risk of voice disorders. The site also has a "frequently asked questions" page about vocal stamina and fatigue, as well as a section on "tips and exercises for getting a great voice."

b. Wake Forest Center for Voice Disorders. http://www.bgsm.edu/voice.

    Plenty of information on laryngopharyngeal reflux and gastroesophageal reflux and voice disorders can be found here. The website contains a special section on singers, singing, and voice disorders, including "10 most common problems of singers" and "medicine in the vocal arts."

c. Pacific Voice Center (British Columbia). http://pvcrp.com. This website advertises training programs for voice care professionals and includes excerpts from Dr. Rammage's book *Vocalizing with Ease* (see section on self-help books later) and how to order it. It has a section on voice amplifiers.

d. Massachusetts Eye and Ear Infirmary Voice Disorder Center.
http://www.voicedisordercenter.meei.harvard.edu.html. Currently being updated.

e. National Center for Voice and Speech. www.ncvs.org. This website has some excellent self-directed "tutorials" on various aspects of voice. The news section is regularly updated. The site provides a link to NCVS's research program on occupational safety in vocalization.

f. The Voice Foundation. www.voicefoundation.org. The official website of the Voice Foundation includes regularly updated information on the Annual Symposium on Care of the Professional Voice. Information on the Journal of Voice and a comprehensive voice care library of relevant papers are available.

General Useful Websites—Gateways to More Specific Sites/Information

a. US National Library of Information.
http://www.nlm.nih.gov/medlineplus/voicedisorders.html.
This site is a means of accessing via the Internet a wide range of professional literature on all aspects of voice and voice disorders.

b. American Academy of Otolaryngology—Head and Neck Surgery http://www.entnet.org/healthinfo.

Click on "throat" and access an excellent range of informative pages about voice production, voice disorders, and self-help voice care issues.

c. American Speech and Hearing Association. http://www.asha.org/public/speech/disorders/Voice-problems.htm.

This public access route to the American Speech and Hearing Association provides information on voice problems, how to identify a voice problem in oneself, and links to professional help (in United States).

d. U.S. National Institute on Deafness and other Communication Disorders. http://www.nidcd.nih.gov.

This site provide more information on voice problems, who and when to contact (in the United States), and self-help advice on voice disorders.

Free publications available at NIDCD http://webdb. nidcd.nih.gov/cgi-bin/dcpubgen.

e. American Laryngological Association. http://www.alahns. org.

Information on upcoming and past meetings as well as a directory of American fellows and officers is available at this site.

f. Society of Otorhinolaryngology and Head–Neck Nurses. www.sohnnurse.com.

This is the site of a national organization of progressive, career-oriented nurses dedicated to professional nursing standards and certification in otorhinolaryngology (ORL) and head–neck nursing.

g. The Voice Academy. www.voiceacademy.org.

The Voice Academy was set up exclusively for the vocal health of US teachers and states that teachers can prevent or self-manage as much as 75% of their voice problems.

h. The Voice Care Network (VCN). http://www.voicecarenet-
    work.org.
    VCN is a nonprofit network of people with a common
    interest in fascinating and engaging but science-based
    voice education. The network's overriding goal is to
    help more and more people enjoy the expressive and
    healthy use of their voices throughout their lives. It
    serves choral conductors, music educators, teachers,
    who take singing classes singers, speech pathologists,
    and ENT physicians. The network's primary mission is
    to use findings from voice sciences as a guide for
    "human-compatible" learning in general music, choral,
    speech, and private voice teaching.

General Health/Medical Resources

a. National Center for Neurogenic Communication Disor-
    ders. http://cnet.shs.arizona.edu. US staff scientists, edu-
    cators, students, and supporting personnel who are
    concerned with speech-and-language disorders caused
    by diseases of the nervous system support this site.

b. National Rehabilitation Information Center. www.naric.
    com (NARIC).
    This site serves anyone, professional or lay person,
    who is interested in disability and rehabilitation,
    including consumers, family members, health profes-
    sionals, educators, rehabilitation counselors, students,
    librarians, administrators, and researchers.

c. Sertoma—(SERvice TO MAnkind) www.sertoma.org.
    Sertoma is a primary service project assisting more
    than 50 million people with speech, hearing, and lan-
    guage disorders.

d. National Institute for Occupational Safety and Health
    (NIOSH). www.cdc.gov/niosh.
    The U.S. federal agency responsible for conducting
    research and making recommendations for the preven-

tion of work-related injury and illness offers information at this site.

RESEARCH-RELATED RESOURCES

Associations

a. Association for Research in Otolaryngology (ARO). www.aro.org.

This international association of scientists and physicians is dedicated to scientific exploration among all of the disciplines in the field of otolaryngology.

b. Council of Academic Programs in Communication Sciences and Disorders. www.capcsd.org. This organization represents academic programs that offer master's, doctoral, and postdoctoral preparation of audiologists, speech-language pathologists, and speech, language, and/or hearing scientists.

Textbooks

a. Mathieson L. The Voice and its Disorders. 6th ed. London: Whurr, 2001.

b. Harris T, Harris S, et al. The Voice Clinic Handbook. London: Whurr, 2000.

c. Dworkin JP, Meleca RJ. Vocal Pathologies: Diagnosis, Treatment, and Case Studies. San Diego: Singular, 1997.

d. Freeman M, Fawcus M. Voice Disorders and their Management. London: Whurr, 2000.

e. Colton RH, Casper JK. Understanding Voice Problems: A Physiological Perspective for Diagnosis and Treatment. 2d ed. Baltimore, MD: Williams and Wilkins, 1996.

f. Gleeson M, ed. Scott and Brown's Otolaryngology and Head and Neck Surgery. 10th ed. Arnold, London. In press.

g. Morrison M, Rammage L. The Management of Voice Disorders. London: Chapman and Hall Medical, 1994.

Self-help Books

a. Martin S, Darnley L. The Teaching Voice. London: Whurr, 1996. ISBN 1-987635-19-2.

b.   Cicely Berry. The Voice and the Actor. London: Harrap, 1991. ISBN 0-245–52021-X.

c.   Cicely Berry. Your Voice and How to Use It. London: Virgin Books, 2003. ISBN 0-86369-826-3.

d.   Bodnitz FS. Keep Your Voice Healthy. College-Hill Press, 1988. ISBN 0-316-109029.

e.   Rodenburg P. The Right to Speak. London: Methuen, 1992. ISBN 0-413-66130-X.

f.   Cornish C. Can You Hear Me at the Back. Bivocal Press, 1995. ISBN 0-9526458-0-7.

g.   Garfield Davies D, Jahn AE. Care of the Professional Voice. Butterworth Heinemann, 1998. ISBN 0-7506-3640-8.

h.   Rammage L. Vocalizing with Ease. British Columbia: Pacific Voice Center, Available via their website (above).

Useful Organizations

a.   The British Voice Association (BVA).
The British Voice Association Institute of Laryngology and Otology, 330 Gray's Inn Road, London, WC1X 8EE, U.K.
Website: http://www.british-voice-association.com.

b.   Voice Care Network UK.
29 Southbank Road, Kenilworth, Warwickshire, CV8 1LA, U.K.
Website: www.voicecare.org.uk.

c.   British Performing Arts Medicine Trust
18 Ogle Street, London, W1P 7LG, U.K.

d.   Royal College of Speech and Language Therapists
2 White Hart Yard, London, SE1 1NX, U.K.
Website: www.rcslt.org.

e.   American Academy of Otolaryngology–Head and Neck Surgery
One Prince Street, Alexandria, Virginia, U.S.A.
E-mail: webmaster@entnet.org. Internet: www.entnet.org.

f. American Laryngological Association (for professionals)
    Montefiore Medical Center, Department of Otolaryngol-
    ogy, 3400 Bainebridge Avenue, 3rd Floor, Bronx, New
    York, U.S.A.
    E-mail: mfried@montefiore.org. Internet: www.alahns.org.

g. American Speech–Language–Hearing Association
    10801 Rockville Pike, Rockville, Maryland, U.S.A.
    E-mail: actioncenter@asha.org. Internet: www.asha.org.

h. Voice Foundation
    1721 Pine Street, Philadelphia, Pennsylvania 19103,
    U.S.A.
    E-mail: voicefound@onrampcom.org. Internet: www. voi-
    cefoundation.org.

i. National Center for Voice and Speech
    University of Iowa, 330 WJSHC, Iowa City, Iowa 52242,
    U.S.A.
    E-mail: webmaster@ncvs.org. Internet: www.ncvs.org.

General Guidance on the Working Environment

a. "General ventilation in the workplace. Guidance for
    employers." HSG202 ISBN 0-7176-1793-9[a].
b. "Thermal comfort in the workplace. Guidance for employ-
    ers." HSG194 ISBN 0-7176-2468-4[a].
c. "Lighting at work HSG38." ISBN 0-7176-1232-5[a].

Specific Guidance on Working in Call Centers

a. Psychosocial Risk Factors in Call Centres: An Evaluation
    of Work Design and Well-Being. Research Report 169.
    Health and Safety Executive 2003[a] (includes findings in
    relation to voice health and a 23-page questionnaire used
    in the study).

---

[a] Priced publications available from HSE Books, P.O. Box 1999, Sudbury,
Suffolk, CO10 2WA, U.K.

Specific Guidance on Occupational Voice Loss

a. Occupational Voice Loss. A Negotiator's Guide. BIFU Research Department. Publication obtainable on 0208 946 9151.

b. "More care for your voice." The Voice Care Network. www.voicecare.org.uk.

Appendix A

Workplace Hazard Checklist for Voice Health

	Yes	No	Action
Environment			
Are the following adequate			
Temperature	☐	☐	–
Humidity	☐	☐	–
Background noise	☐	☐	–
Dust/cleanliness	☐	☐	–
Ergonomic arrangement of workstation	☐	☐	–
Lighting			
Generally	☐	☐	–
For specific tasks	☐	☐	–
Smoke free	☐	☐	–

This document is not intended to replace the need for professional advice which should be sought from a competent advisor

	Yes	No	Action
Availability of water	☐	☐	—
Work			
Is the work designed			
To include breaks	☐	☐	—
To reduce overuse with clients	☐	☐	—
To reduce overuse with colleagues	☐	☐	—
To consider vocal demands			
when it is designed or changed?	☐	☐	—
Workers			
Are workers informed about voice health			
During induction	☐	☐	—
On change of jobs	☐	☐	—
Are they encouraged to report			
symptoms early?	☐	☐	—

Checklist completed by:

Name:

Role:

Date:

Actions for completion by whom:

Actions to be completed by when:

Date for review:

Appendix B

Suggested Sample Training Program for Voice Users

Content

1. Why voice health is important
2. How the voice is produced
3. What causes voice problems (at work, socially, and at home)
4. What can go wrong: the symptoms and signs
5. Prevention (rest, avoid overuse, humidity, hydration, etc.)
6. The company policy (duties and responsibilities of those concerned) and importance of early reporting (what symptoms to report, to whom, and when)
7. What your manager will do if you report symptoms (request details of complaint, seek alternative tasks if one or more is

---

This document is not intended to replace the need for professional advice which should be sought from a competent advisor

felt to be too difficult, review, involve occupational health resources if needed)
8. What happens if serious problems develop (refer to company policy on capability)
9. Reviewing your current work activity and reducing risks (encourage employees to participate and address problems themselves, informally)

Appendix C

Sample Company Policy on Voice Health

Introduction

The company takes the issue of employee health seriously and initiates steps to prevent ill health from work. We recognize that individuals may have medical conditions that directly affect their voice or may need to take medication for unrelated conditions that may affect their ability to do their job because of voice problems.

This policy sets out the roles and responsibilities of individuals, managers, and advisors, and describes the action to be taken with respect to voice problems.

This document is not intended to replace the need for professional advice which should be sought from a competent advisor

Statement

The company aims to prevent occupational voice disorders and minimize the consequences should they already exist. The company will design work and work activities to support voice health and will adapt work, if possible, to reduce the risks of voice ill health. This policy should be read in conjunction with the general health and safety and human resources policies.

Roles and Responsibilities

Directors

Role

The directors' role is to ensure that the company policy is adequately resourced and that its compliance is monitored.

Responsibility

They remain responsible for the health of their employees. For example, Mr. John Smith, Director of Human Resources, is responsible for health and safety at Board level.

Line Managers

Role

Line managers/supervisors' role is to ensure awareness of the voice health policy, the risks of developing voice disorders, and the actions to be taken to prevent and manage them.

Responsibility

Line managers are responsible for

1. Ensuring that risk assessments are undertaken,
2. Actions that are carried out to control risks,
3. Ensuring the cases of voice problems are brought to the attention of the directors, and
4. Employees attending the necessary training and being aware of early reporting arrangements.

Employees

Role

The employees' role is to follow company policies in carrying out their work and work with their managers to create a healthy and safe workplace.

Responsibility

Employees are responsible for

1. Abiding by the company policy,
2. Reporting symptoms early to their line manager, and
3. Reporting problems with the working environment promptly.

Human Resources

Role

The company HR function will support employees and line managers in following the company policy and will access specialist support as needed.

Responsibility

HR is responsible for identifying and arranging suitable training courses and specialist occupational health advice. It is also responsible for advising the company and employee on its personnel policies and procedures and managing performance issues related to ill health.

Occupational Health

Role

The role of Occupational Health is to support the business and the employee and provide professional advice on the prevention and management of ill health.

Responsibility

Occupational Health is responsible for providing specialist advice on voice ill health prevention at the work design stage and to employer and employee should problems occur.

Appendix D

Short Questionnaire for Assessment of Voice Symptoms in a Working Population

CONFIDENTIAL
VOICE HEALTH QUESTIONNAIRE

1. Name (optional) _____

2. Gender   Male ☐   Female ☐

3. Date of birth _____

4. Time working in this type of job _____ years _____ months

5. Job title _____

6. Have you ever had any training or information on looking after your voice?   Yes ☐   No ☐

This document is not intended to replace the need for professional advice which should be sought from a competent advisor

7. Have you had or do you have (check one or more)

	Now	In last 3 months	More than 3 months ago
Hoarseness	☐	☐	☐
Tired voice	☐	☐	☐
Loss of voice	☐	☐	☐
Dry throat	☐	☐	☐
Sore throat	☐	☐	☐
Effort needed to speak	☐	☐	☐
Feeling of spasm in voice	☐	☐	☐
High speaking voice	☐	☐	☐
Low speaking voice	☐	☐	☐
Difficulty with high notes	☐	☐	☐
Need to cough/clear throat	☐	☐	☐

If you have checked any of the above, go to question 8. If you have not checked any of the above, go to question 11.

8. For each of the problems below, check the number that best describes how big a problem it was for you.

	No problem				Major problem
I have/had trouble speaking loudly or being heard in noisy situations	1	2	3	4	5
I run/ran out of air and need to take frequent breaths when talking	1	2	3	4	5
I am/was sometimes anxious or frustrated (because of my voice)	1	2	3	4	5
I sometimes get/got depressed (because of my voice)	1	2	3	4	5
I have/had trouble using the telephone (because of my voice)	1	2	3	4	5
I have/had trouble doing my job or practicing my profession (because of my voice)	1	2	3	4	5
I avoid/avoided going out socially (because of my voice)	1	2	3	4	5
I have/had to repeat myself to be understood	1	2	3	4	5
I have/had become less outgoing (because of my voice)	1	2	3	4	5

How many sick days have you had in the last year because
of your voice? _____days
How many days did you have on alternative job?

_____days

9. Did your voice problem start following

		Yes	No
9.1.	Surgery	☐	☐
9.2.	A respiratory infection	☐	☐
9.3.	Trauma	☐	☐
9.4.	Increased use of your voice	☐	☐
9.5.	Anything else _____	☐	☐

_____

_____

10. Was your voice problem

		Yes	No
10.1.	Caused by your work	☐	☐
10.2.	Aggravated by your work	☐	☐
10.3.	Unrelated to your work	☐	☐
10.4.	Caused by your hobbies	☐	☐
10.5.	Aggravated by your hobbies	☐	☐
10.6.	Unrelated to your hobbies	☐	☐

If you have answered yes to 10.4, 10.5, or 10.6, please list
your hobbies:

11. Is there anything you would like to add?

Thank you for completing this questionnaire.

Index

Abduction, 2–3
Accelerometers, 56
Acoustic signal, 5
Aerodynamic measurements, 48
Amplitude, 5, 57
Ary-epiglottic folds, 2
Arytenoid cartilages, 2
Association for Research in
    Otolaryngology (ARO), 100

Background noise, 54, 81, 105
Breath flow. See Transglottic
    air flow
Breathing patterns, 30
Breath support, 33, 74
British Voice Association (BVA),
    102
Bronchodilators, 71,

Cavities, 5
  nasal, 5
  oral, 5
  pharyngeal, 5
Chemical agents, 36
Chronic sinusitis, 33

Clinical science
  voice misuse, 34
Claims, 89
  occupational damages, 89
Council of Academic Programs in
    Communication Sciences
    and Disorders, 101

Disability Discrimination Act 1995
    (DDA), 85–86
Dosimeters, 55–56
Dysphonia, 29, 35–37
  functional, 95
  work-induced, 93

Etiology, 25–44
Endocrinological disorders, 26–27
Endoscopic examination, 35, 48
Environmental conditions, 36, 38

Formaldehyde, 36–38
Frequency, 4
  fundamental, 55
  high, 14
  low, 12